11/17

RANDOM HOUSE

LARGE
PRINT

Also by Arthur Agatston, M.D.
available from Random House Large Print

The South Beach Diet

THE SOUTH BEACH DIET
Cookbook

Arthur Agatston, M.D.

Author of *The South Beach Diet*

RANDOM HOUSE LARGE PRINT

© 2004 by Arthur Agatston, M.D.

Recipes on pages 51, 58, 62, 68, 73, 76, 78, 79, 80, 86, 90, 93, 102, 105, 112, 118, 119, 128, 135, 143, 146, 157, 159, 164, 179, 185, 190, 193, 197, 198, 200, 203, 212, 213, 215, 216, 217, 220, 222, 223, 225, 226, 248, 261, 262, 275, 277, 285, 290, 296, 299, 301, 315, 320, 331, 333, 341, 357, 368, 370, 373, 375, 377, 384, 389, 392, 418, 431, 440, 442, 446, 449, 450, 453, 470, 471, 473, 478, 480, 485 remain © Rodale Inc.

Photographs © 2004 by Rodale Inc.

All rights reserved under International and Pan-American Copyright Conventions. Published in the United States of America by Random House Large Print in association with Rodale Inc., New York and simultaneously in Canada by Random House of Canada Limited, Toronto. Distributed by Random House, Inc., New York.

Book design by Carol Angstadt
Food styling by Diane Vezza
Prop styling by Melissa DeMayo
Photography by Mitch Mandel

The Library of Congress has established a Cataloging-in-Publication record for this title

0-375-43343-0

www.randomlargeprint.com

FIRST LARGE PRINT EDITION

10 9 8 7 6 5 4 3 2 1

This Large Print edition published in accord with the standards of the N.A.V.H.

For my sons, Evan and Adam, who have

always been interested and enthusiastic supporters

of my work. My wish is that you, too, find

passion and satisfaction in your chosen professions.

And, as always, to my wife and partner, Sari,

for her counsel, her support, and her love.

ACKNOWLEDGMENTS

First and foremost, I'd like to thank my patients and all the followers of *The South Beach Diet*. You helped make the first book a tremendous success, and your ideas and feedback have been invaluable. In addition, your continued enthusiasm has helped promote the important national discussion about healthy eating.

A very special thank you to my wife, Sari, who worked long and hard on the creation of this book and to Marie Almon, our nutritionist, for her tremendous help developing recipes and overseeing the nutritional aspect of the project.

My editor, Margot Schupf, has been a real partner in this effort and a delight to work with. Jennifer Reich, Carol Angstadt, Mitch Mandel, and Diane Vezza were especially instrumental on the design and production side of things. I would also like to acknowledge and thank the entire team at Rodale, including Tami Booth, Amy Rhodes, Cindy Ratzlaff, and Cathy Gruhn. Another note of thanks to Lee Brian Schrager and Terry Zarikian for their help in bringing the great chefs of South Beach to this project.

And finally, thanks to Heidi Krupp, my publicist, for her tremendous enthusiasm, and to Richard Pine, my literary agent, for his sound advice and friendship.

CONTENTS

INTRODUCTION

The South Beach Diet was made for people who love to eat.

That will be obvious to anyone who pays attention to current trends in cooking and eating. But you don't have to be a gourmet chef to know what I'm talking about—it's evident in every restaurant menu, every magazine and newspaper article, every cooking show on TV about how we eat now. Today's best cuisines make use of a wide variety of fresh, wholesome, delicious foods prepared in exciting ways.

Similarly, the South Beach Diet encourages you to eat a great variety of foods and to cook them in a healthy manner. On this diet, you can have abundant quantities of nearly any kind of meat or fish you can name. Vegetables and fruits, too. And because the South Beach program is neither low-carb nor low-fat, you'll be enjoying many of the dishes that other diets require you to give up completely. On our plan, you will eat meals that fully satisfy your hunger; you are even urged to have between-meal snacks and desserts. The types of recipes we offer in this book could be found in any popular cookbook.

Another reason why I say this diet is for food lovers is because of one of its main principles: that we've become an overweight society because we eat too many processed foods. These contain the "bad" carbohydrates—such as white flour or white sugar—where much of the digestion has begun in factories instead of in our stomachs. This causes our bodies to store excess fat, especially around our midsections. Plus, eating these bad carbs creates cravings for more unhealthy foods; instead of simply satisfying our hunger, they actually make it worse. Eating fewer processed carbohydrates and more dishes made from good, wholesome ingredients will almost automatically bring about weight loss and improved overall health. You'll eat well, too—maybe better than you have in a long time. That's another good reason for a South Beach cookbook. I hope that once you've tried some of the recipes, you'll agree.

As I write this, *The South Beach Diet*, based on the eating plan I developed, is atop the national bestseller lists. Later in this book, I will explain the diet itself and how it came to exist. For now, suffice it to say that the program grew out of my concerns as a cardiologist for the health and well-being of my patients.

If you're already familiar with the South Beach Diet, you'll know that the diet is divided into three phases. To help make things easy for you, every recipe in this book is marked to indicate a phase of the diet—recipes marked as Phase 1 can be enjoyed from the very beginning. Recipes marked as Phase 2 can be enjoyed after you've reached that point in the diet. And Phase 3 recipes are for when you've fully integrated the diet into your lifestyle. There are also 25 recipes from prominent chefs that will make your mouth water. And they all fit into the diet!

Another feature of this book is the shopping list

beginning on page 22. This will help you decide what to buy at the supermarket, and what to leave behind. Check out "Ask Dr. Agatston" on page 35 to find the answers to the questions asked most frequently about the South Beach Diet. Also included are real-life South Beach success stories and tips from people who have shared their motivating stories on the South Beach message boards at www.prevention.com. I hope they will inspire you to achieve your own success.

The diet has succeeded far beyond my expectations. It is responsible for millions of Americans losing weight safely and easily, and keeping it off while also improving their blood chemistries. My goal is to extend the benefits of the South Beach Diet to still more Americans. There are several ways to accomplish this. I have observed the best long-term results in those who have a good understanding of the few basic principles of the diet. This allows them to use flexibility and good judgment when making food choices in the various eating situations we all face: during travel, parties, stress, fatigue, and when dining out. The other factor responsible for long-term compliance is the variety of foods and recipes available. This combats the repetition that leads to boredom on so many diets. Our goal for our heart patients as well as all of our readers is an overall healthier lifestyle leading to many permanent benefits.

In the meantime, I hope this cookbook helps you find the quality and variety of dishes to enable you to make the South Beach Diet the lifestyle it was intended to be.

WHAT IS THE SOUTH BEACH DIET?

Enjoying good food is a pleasure.

Eating is necessary for survival, of course, but it is also one of the great joys of life. We so love eating that we give our meals a social function. We enjoy our families and friendships around tables laden with good things to eat.

But our pleasure has also become our peril. Our relationship with food—or, rather, our excessive appetites for certain foods—is today, in many cases, hazardous to our health. If you've read the news magazines and periodicals recently, you know what I'm talking about—skyrocketing obesity, which is associated with heart disease, cancer, strokes, and diabetes, as a result of our unhealthy eating habits.

For years, we were taught by the experts that maintaining proper weight required sacrifice—that the only way to stay lean and mean was to give up many of the foods we loved. Millions of us started that challenging journey to good health but didn't necessarily get there. Many popular diets are geared to short-term weight loss and are clearly inappropriate for long-term weight control. In contrast, the South Beach Diet was developed to prevent heart attacks and strokes by improving our blood chemistries and trimming our waistlines. This means adopting a healthy lifestyle, not just looking for a quick fix.

Finding the *Real* Problem

Why has there been so much confusion about diet? It has largely been because through new research, new information has been brought to light that has changed the conventional wisdom on how our bodies process food. The important effects of fiber, the glycemic index (how fast a food raises our blood sugar), the good fats, and the syndrome of pre-diabetes on weight and on health were simply not appreciated until recently.

But diets also failed because they didn't take into account how the average human being operates. The weight loss regimens were often impractical, cumbersome, unnatural, and severe. They required us to abandon forever the joys of eating a wide variety of good foods in amounts sufficient to satisfy our hunger and please our tastebuds.

I had a front-row view of how our misconceptions about nutrition and weight loss led us astray. As a cardiologist, my primary interest has been the prevention of heart disease. My proudest achievement thus far has been my role in the development of a heart scan protocol that uses electron beam computerized tomography (EBT) scan technology—which can, in minutes, easily and painlessly detect the buildup of arteriosclerosis in the walls of arteries years before it causes a heart attack or stroke. Around the world, the measure of coronary calcium (or plaque, as you might know it) is referred to as the Agatston Score.

That technology has saved many lives by detecting problems that would otherwise go unseen and finding them early enough to treat them without surgery. While this test can detect problems early, it cannot in itself prevent heart disease. But lifestyle changes, including proper diet and exercise, as well as certain medications, can prevent heart attacks. In this realm, I was stymied. Like other cardiologists, I urged my patients to lose weight and cut their cholesterol levels by going on the low-fat diet prescribed by the American Heart Association and other experts. But it didn't work as planned. Some patients went the low-fat route but didn't lose much weight at all. A few would diet religiously and exercise as they were instructed, lose the extra pounds, and feel fine. But then they'd grow tired of always feeling hungry, or they'd miss their favorite foods, or their willpower would just wear down. At that point, they'd start cheating here and there, and before we knew it, all the excess weight was back. In many cases, they'd end up heavier than before they started to diet. Too-rapid weight loss associated with crash diets actually lowers our metabolism and predisposes us to yo-yo dieting. In fact, the failures of low-fat, high-carb plans as well as rapid weight loss strategies have been well-documented in study after study.

Despite the lack of scientific proof that it worked, the low-fat regimen became our national weight loss gospel. We were lectured about the evils of meat, eggs, cheese, even salad oil. In response, food manufacturers began developing an entirely new category of products labeled "low-fat" or "low-cholesterol," which included everything from cookies and hot dogs to salad dressing and potato chips. The foods *were* lower in fats or cholesterol, just as advertised. There was just one problem: The fats and/or cholesterol had been replaced by "processed" carbohydrates—various forms of sugar for the most part, either white sugar itself or high fructose corn syrup, honey, molasses, and starches bereft of fiber and nutrients.

In response, people felt free to eat these products with gusto. Unfortunately, I was one of those people consuming low-fat goodies whole hog—what a mistake! We had no idea that we were taking in more sugars and starches than ever before, and that this was causing rapid, large swings in our blood sugars that made us hungry again soon after we finished a meal or a snack. The national—and now international—epidemic of obesity and diabetes was the result.

The "Good Fats"

Because of my frustration with the low-fat, high-carb approach, and because I witnessed some successes with other high-saturated-fat, low-carb diets, I began my own study of the nutrition and weight loss literature. I wanted to find a healthy eating plan I could offer to my patients, something that would allow them to eat well but also to lose weight and improve their blood chemistries.

It soon became clear that the low-fat plan was fatally flawed. The bad fats—the so-called saturated ones, which exist mainly in animal products such as fatty meats, butter, cream, and cheeses—*did* contribute to obesity, to some extent. But not nearly as much as we had been led to think. Their main health hazard was that they contributed to high cholesterol and triglycerides, which in turn led to cardiovascular disease. As a cardiologist, that concerned me.

But there are also good fats, in particular, the Mediterranean oils, including extra virgin olive oil, canola oil, omega-3 fish oils, and the oils found in most nuts. These fats are not bad. They are not neutral. They are actually good for us. They help prevent heart attacks and strokes and also help our sugar and insulin metabolism, leading to better long-term weight control.

The "Good Carbs"

As I studied, I learned that just as you cannot lump all fats together, neither can you lump together all carbohydrates. Just as there are good fats and bad fats, there are also good carbs and bad carbs. More precisely, there is a whole spectrum of carbohydrates from very bad, to not so bad, to pretty good, and finally, very good. A well-rounded diet makes good use of good carbs.

There has never been any question about the benefits of eating carbs such as vegetables, beans, and fruits. But back when the anti-fat gospel still held sway, we were instructed that even the starchiest refined carbohydrates—white bread, white pasta, potatoes, and instant rice—were healthy. In fact, however, these foods undermined our best efforts to lose weight.

All carbohydrates, even the healthiest vegetables, contain sugars. Starches, such as those found in potatoes, rice, and wheat flour, are merely chains of sugar molecules. In the course of digestion, our bodies extract those sugars and put them to good use, providing us with necessary energy. Without sugars, we would die.

But before we can access those sugars, our digestive systems must separate them from the fiber that carbs also contain. That fiber slows down the digestive process, which is a good thing. It means that the sugars are released gradually into our bloodstreams. When that happens, the pancreas gets the signal and begins producing insulin. It is insulin's job to transport that blood sugar into our cells, where it can be burned for immediate energy or stored for later use.

Something very different takes place when we eat carbs that contain little or none of their original fiber, however. When that happens, our digestive systems begin processing all the sugars rapidly. As a result, the level of blood sugar—glucose—rises sharply, prompting the pancreas to release a large amount of insulin at once. In fact, the pancreas may actually overreact and send forth more insulin than is needed. That, in turn, causes a sharp drop in the level of glucose.

You are unaware of all this happening inside your body, but the fact is that you do sense it in an indirect way. That dramatic rise and fall of blood sugar creates cravings for more food. Your hunger is merely a response to changes in blood chemistry brought about by your metabolism. This particular sensation drives you to want more food sooner than you would otherwise desire. And the craving is for more carbs.

The propensity of a food to cause swings in blood sugar is known as the glycemic index (GI). It was developed in the 1980s by David Jenkins, M.D., Ph.D., of the University of Toronto. This important concept was not available to the developers of earlier diets. The GI is a system that ranks foods by how quickly they cause blood sugar to rise when tested against 50 grams of glucose, which has a GI of 100. If the GI of food X is 50 percent, then it raises blood sugar only 50 percent as fast as glucose does. While we always assumed that table sugar raises your blood sugar faster than a white potato, Dr. Jenkins's glycemic index taught us that it doesn't. Why is this so important? The faster your blood sugar goes up after a meal, the faster it falls. In fact, after high-glycemic-index meals, your blood sugar is likely to peak rapidly and then dive to a level lower than where it started. This blood sugar roller coaster results in a range of feelings including irresistible cravings, severe fatigue, sleepiness, headaches, and anxiety.

Once this phenomenon—known as reactive hypoglycemia—occurs, you will typically grab the first carbohydrates available that will raise your blood sugar. Because the foods that raise your blood sugar the fastest are the ones that relieve your symptoms the fastest, they are what you reach for. This kicks off a vicious cycle. It takes time for your body to recognize that its blood sugar levels have normalized, but during this period you continue eating because you don't yet feel satisfied. So, without realizing it, you overeat, which leads to further swings in blood sugar, and the cycle repeats. This pattern is responsible for America's epidemic of obesity and diabetes.

These facts of human metabolism have always been true. But the way our bodies process food is at odds with the market's emphasis on quick, convenient, and easy cooking. Virtually all of the fiber has been removed from everything made from white flour, for instance. That means most commercially made breads, crackers, and muffins—anything that is baked. The same is true for breakfast cereals, even some of those that claim to be healthy, such as instant oatmeal. All sweets fall under this category, too—cakes, cookies, doughnuts, and the rest. Pancakes and waffles as well. Even rice has been processed for easy cooking—the removal of the fiber is why it can be ready so quickly.

Fiber contains important vitamins and minerals, and when you remove fiber, you remove those nutrients as well. This is why these carbs have been called "empty calories." Other than calories, they give us nothing else that our bodies require for optimal functioning. The fiber is also the element that slows the digestion of the carbohydrates. It encourages a slow, steady supply of sugar (energy) to our bodies, allowing us to function well for long periods without symptoms of hypoglycemia.

Reversing the Trend

How do we reverse the obesity epidemic? We adopt a diet of good carbs with plenty of natural vitamins and nutrients and good, healthy fats. In other words, we adopt the South Beach Diet.

As I mentioned, bad carbs are everywhere. They go into the most convenient foods, all the snacks that have become such a ubiquitous part of contemporary eating. Some people have a weakness for salty snacks, such as potato chips or pretzels, which contain lots of bad carbs. Others have a nagging sweet tooth driving them to eat chocolate, ice cream, or baked goods. Some people are beset by cravings for bread, pasta, potatoes, or rice. Whatever the craving, the result is the same: We overwhelm our systems with frequent infusions of highly processed carbohydrates and, in turn, our bodies respond with urges for more. It's a strange phenomenon in that the food we eat, rather than satisfying our hunger, actually creates more hunger of its own.

Once this physiology became clear, an anti-carbohydrate camp rose up among some diet experts. Suddenly, all carbs were being blamed as the primary cause of obesity. In truth, a diet that's too low in carbohydrates will be lacking in nutrients, natural vitamins, and dietary fiber—all of which are necessary for optimal health.

What's more, people enjoy eating carbohydrates. To give up foods such as bread, pasta, rice, and even fruits and some vegetables seemed to be a terrible mistake. And by this point, we had all suffered enough under weight loss plans that required us to give up foods we loved. It is possible to eat carbs, even bread and rice and so on, as long as the grains have not been overly processed. If the whole grain is still present, carbs can be eaten by people watching their weight.

If you eat the right fats, like the kind found in olive oil, nuts, avocados, and omega-3 fish oils, you can still lose weight and improve your health. And, good fats make our food taste good. That's another reason they're such an integral part of the South Beach Diet.

The South Beach Diet: Striking the Balance

This was when it dawned on me that a healthy diet would be neither low-fat nor low-carb. Those extremes had caused, rather than cured, our obesity problem. A sound weight loss plan would make the distinction between good and bad fats and carbs. It would allow dieters to eat enough of the good ones so that no one would really miss the bad.

That was the first principle of the South Beach Diet.

The diet would make ample use of the foods that taste good and satisfy hunger: meats, poultry, seafood, and vegetables, all cooked using good fats such as extra virgin olive oil and made flavorful with the right sauces and spices.

Another principle was that the food would have to be served in portions large enough to satisfy normal hunger.

No one can go through life constantly feeling hunger pangs. That's why the South Beach Diet suggests strategic snacking throughout the day.

As a chocoholic, I understand the importance of dessert. Because the South Beach Diet is meant to allow you to eat as naturally as possible, it includes desserts, even in the strictest phase. I think we've included some excellent dessert recipes in this book—dishes that taste great but can be enjoyed without falling off the weight loss wagon. Many of the dessert recipes are fruit-based and replace sugar with a no-calorie sugar substitute. When possible, the fats are healthy ones rather than the saturated fats or trans fats that can lead to health problems.

As those who have read *The South Beach Diet* are aware, the program is structured into three phases. The first, most restrictive, phase lasts for 2 weeks. It eliminates all starches including breads, rice, pasta, and baked goods. It also restricts sugars, including all fruits and—sorry folks—allows no alcohol. You stay on Phase 2 until you reach your target weight. You add back starches in the form of whole grains, sugars in the form of low-glycemic fruits, and alcohol with meals. Once you've reached your goal weight, you begin the third phase, which is maintenance. At this point, the diet has become a lifestyle—a new way of eating that permits you to have the foods you like and still maintain your health and keep the weight off. You remain aware of what you learned in the first two phases, choosing a sweet potato instead of a white potato, brown rice instead of white, and whole grain bread instead of white bread. In other words, you have learned the pecking order of the various classes of carbohydrates and how to apply it to your everyday life.

An important key to turning the South Beach Diet from a diet program into a lifestyle is to have a great variety of foods and recipes that are simple and delicious. This cookbook will provide you with more than 200 choices to keep your meals fresh and exciting.

Here's to your health and bon appétit!

STOCKING THE SOUTH BEACH DIET KITCHEN

Changing how you eat will require some changes in how you shop, too. In fact, it will transform your kitchen, because that is the arena where dieters either succeed or fail. (I was going to say it's where you win or lose, except that in this particular contest, when you lose, you win!) Anyway, your pantry, refrigerator, and freezer should look quite a bit different—vastly improved, of course—once you're on the South Beach Diet.

I can't emphasize enough the importance of having the right foods around the house, and not having the wrong ones. When I talk to people who have wavered on the diet, I hear the same basic story over and over: "I got home from work late, I was starving, and there were no vegetables in the refrigerator—so I microwaved a bag of frozen french fries instead." Or, "There was no sugar-free gelatin dessert, so I had a cupcake." Or, "I ran out of almonds so I ate some pretzels, washed down with a soda." The South Beach Diet allows you a wide variety of delicious foods. You won't have to count calories or measure the quantities you consume. But it is important to steer clear of the truly unhealthy items that will undermine your success.

Even when you try, it's not always going to be the easiest thing to do. For example, when one member of a couple goes on the diet and the other does not, a simple thing like a loaf of bread can become a battle-ground—the dieter wishes it would disappear, while the partner needs it for his or her daily sandwich. In one household I know, the wife has banished all bread, and the husband now goes out every afternoon to buy a single fresh roll for lunch. Dieters with children have an especially challenging time—no parent wants to deprive the kids of their little treats, but you may find it impossible to resist raiding the cookie jar yourself. Willpower is needed, of course, though if you can get the children to love no-sugar-added fudge pops, you'll all be better off.

Maintaining a South Beach Diet–friendly kitchen is imperative if you're going to adopt healthy eating habits and lose excess weight. This chapter is a guide to what groceries you'll need to buy before you begin the diet. The list contains foods that are acceptable in Phase 1—the initial, strict phase—and also in Phases 2 and 3, the less restrictive stages. I want to help you to create a healthy, balanced, well-appointed kitchen—a place where you can eat well *and* lose weight in the coming weeks or months.

You don't need to go out and buy every single item listed here; let your personal tastes be your guide. Your goal should be simply to stock up on the foods you like to eat. If you fill up on good foods, you won't have the need (or even the room) for anything else. Everything here should be available in any well-stocked supermarket. If you can't find a particular item where you shop, you can skip it and replace it with something else.

Cleaning Out the Pantry

Before you start that shopping trip, however, you may need to clear some space in your kitchen. So first, go through your pantry, refrigerator, and freezer and rid them of the foods that do not fit in the South Beach Diet. Some items can be packed away during the first 2 weeks on the diet, after which they will be allowed once more. Other goodies—the really troublesome ones—should probably just vanish forever. After the first phase of the diet, I promise, you will not miss them.

The list that follows contains many of the foods that you'll need to eliminate during Phase 1 of the South

Beach Diet as well as some foods that are off-limits for Phase 2 as well. The list is very comprehensive, but it's impossible to list every food that dieters should avoid. Here's one good rule of thumb: If, among the first three ingredients, you see sugar in any form—meaning sugar itself or fructose, maltose, dextrose, or anything with the suffix -*ose*—that food is almost certainly off-limits. During Phase 1, anything made with flour is taboo. After that, anything made with enriched white flour is off-limits. Whole wheat flour is better for you, but even then, you should not be eating baked goods with less than 3 grams of dietary fiber per serving.

So before you start Phase 1 of the diet, go through your kitchen and remove the following items:

Baked goods: This means all breads, cakes, crackers, cookies, cupcakes, pastries, and waffles. Even the healthiest breads made with whole wheat flour must go away during Phase 1. Muffins as well—English and otherwise.

Beverages: All fruit juices are banned for the first 2 weeks of the plan. All sodas and any other drinks containing sugar, fructose, or corn syrup are also forbidden.

Also for Phase 1, all alcoholic beverages are off-limits. That includes beer, premixed cocktails, whiskey, wine, and wine coolers.

Cereals: All varieties of cereals are off-limits during the first 2 weeks of the diet. That includes the healthy ones high in fiber and with no added sugar, like oat bran and kashi. The carbs in many commercial cereals cause a steep rise in blood sugar, which creates cravings for more carbs. Healthy high-fiber cereals reappear in Phase 2.

Condiments, dressings, and seasonings: Barbecue sauce, honey mustard, ketchup, and any other condiment or sauce made with corn syrup, molasses, or sugar is banned. Even low-fat or fat-free condiments, such as barbecue sauces, mayonnaise, salad dressings, and the like are also off-limits. Surprised? In these products, the fat is usually replaced by refined carbohydrates.

Most commercial teriyaki sauce is also forbidden because of its sugar content. Sweet pickles and relish are also banned.

Get rid of any commercially made salad dressing that contains sugars (including fructose) or carbs, fat-free dressings included. Dressings made with extra virgin olive oil and vinegar are fine. No-carb, sugar-free dressings are okay as well.

Dairy: Whole milk is banned in all phases of the South Beach Diet because of the saturated fats it contains. Cheeses made with anything but 2% milk or part-skim or fat-free milk are also off-limits in Phase 1. No brie or other creamy cheeses for sure. Butter is severely limited.

Fish and shellfish: There's no need to get rid of any fish. All fish are okay, canned or fresh. The oily ones—anchovies, mackerel, salmon, and sardines—are especially recommended for the healthy omega-3 oils they contain.

Flour: All flour is taboo for Phase 1. Same for pancake or waffle mix. Cornmeal is also not permitted.

Fruit: All fruit is forbidden during Phase 1. You'll reintroduce fruits to your diet 2 weeks from now, but until then, they have to go. Not only do they contain a lot of sugar, but they stimulate hunger, too. Same for any fruit products—jellies, jams, and dried fruits, including raisins. Of course, any frozen foods containing fruit or fruit juice are also forbidden during Phase 1.

Meat and poultry: The South Beach Diet makes plentiful use of meat and poultry, but certain ones are off-limits. Anything processed using sugars—honey-baked or maple-cured ham, for instance—is forbidden on all phases. Most luncheon meats are allowed, but when buying packaged products, be sure to check the ingredients. If you find any form of sugar in there, put it back.

During Phase 1, fatty fowl such as duck and goose shouldn't be on the menu. Pâté is forbidden, too. Dark-meat chicken or turkey (legs and wings) are higher in fat and cholesterol and also are not allowed. Any processed fowl, such as packaged chicken nuggets or patties, are forbidden in all phases. Bacon and breakfast sausage are both off-limits in all phases due to the saturated fats.

Get rid of any beef brisket, liver, rib steaks, or other fatty cuts. Same goes for veal breast.

Oils and fats: As you clean out your kitchen, get rid of any solid vegetable shortening or lard.

Pasta: Any kind of pasta is gone for Phase 1, even whole wheat.

Rice: Rice of all varieties, even brown, is off-limits for the first 2 weeks.

Snacks: All packaged snacks are off-limits, both the salty variety (cheese puffs, popcorn, potato chips, pretzels, taco chips, and so on) and the sweet kind (cupcakes, cookies, and the rest).

If we could just cut all processed foods from our diet, our weight would drop, and our overall health would improve. Where weight loss is concerned, processed carbs are problematic because the fiber, minerals, and vitamins have been removed.

The type of carbs in these salty or sweet snacks causes a steep rise in blood sugar, which creates cravings for more carbs. Processed carbs are often labeled as "fortified" or "vitamin-enriched" because of the manufacturers' attempt to restore some of the lost nutrients. But you can't replace natural vitamins with artificial ones and get the same health benefits. And many commercially prepared snack foods contain trans fats.

Soup: Rid your kitchen of all powdered soup mixes for the first 2 weeks, because many are full of trans fats. You can have reduced-fat canned bean or clear broth soups in any phase.

Sweeteners: All sweeteners, except sugar substitutes, are off-limits in Phase 1. This includes white sugar, brown sugar, honey, molasses, and corn syrup.

Vegetables: Believe it or not, even a few vegetables must go for Phase 1. Potatoes are the biggest no-no—even boiled. Your digestive system immediately breaks the starches down into sugars, which end up as stored excess weight. Potatoes also create cravings for more bad carbs. This includes white potatoes, but also sweet potatoes and yams.

Corn is also forbidden for now, along with beets, butternut squash, and acorn squash. All are turned quickly into sugars and stimulate hunger pangs. Even carrots are out of bounds for the first 2 weeks. Go through your freezer and get rid of any packaged frozen foods that contain these vegetables.

The South Beach Shopping List

These are the items you're encouraged to enjoy on the South Beach Diet. I've broken this list into two sections. The first details the foods to enjoy in Phase 1, the most restrictive 2 weeks of the diet. The second lists the foods to eat in Phase 2.

You don't need a list for Phase 3. This is how you'll eat for the rest of your life, and you'll know enough about the plan to make the right choices.

Phase 1 Shopping

Baked goods: Steer clear of all baked goods during the entire 2 weeks of Phase 1.

Beverages: Regular, caffeinated coffee is allowed, but no more than 2 cups a day, because caffeine has been found to stimulate insulin production. Decaf is permitted without limits. Tea is allowed, with the same qualifications.

Obviously, water is fine. Flavored waters are all right, too, as long as they don't have calories. Check the labels to be sure. Club soda and seltzer are okay. If you prefer the flavored kinds, check the ingredients to make sure there's no sugar added.

Diet sodas and low-calorie iced teas and powdered drinks are all fine. Some dieters who love orange juice with breakfast replace it with low-cal powdered orange drinks, such as the one from Crystal Light. V8 juice or a similar vegetable cocktail juice is allowed.

Cereals: No cereals are allowed in Phase 1.

Condiments, dressings, and seasonings: Stock up on all spices that contain no added sugar. Extracts, such as almond and vanilla, are great to add to your foods as well. Any kind of pepper is fine, too: black, cayenne, red, and white.

Just about any spice or seasoning is fine on this diet. In fact, I encourage you to use anything you like that enhances the flavor of food. If your healthy dishes taste great, you'll be less tempted to indulge in the unhealthy ones. Why not try the myriad spices and seasonings available in your grocery store?

Try standards like basil, oregano, and parsley, or add a

little heat with cumin, curry, or red pepper. Garlic is something you'll get lots of use from—you can buy it fresh, powdered, or minced. Nutmeg, cinnamon (ground, not cinnamon-sugar!), and cloves will add a cozy warmth to a dish, while dill, mint, and rosemary will add a striking freshness. Used alone or in combination, seasonings will breathe new life into any dish you make.

Any mustard (except honey mustard), mayonnaise (regular, not fat-free), chimichurri steak sauce, hot sauce or Tabasco, prepared horseradish, salsa, light (low-sodium) soy sauce, or Worcestershire sauce is legal in all phases, even 1. See the recipes beginning on page 239 for some homemade condiments you'll love.

To dress your salads, choose any of the approved oils (such as canola, flaxseed, extra virgin olive oil, peanut, sesame, or walnut) mixed with vinegar (such as balsamic or wine). Among the prepared dressings, Newman's Own Light Balsamic Vinaigrette or Newman's Own Olive Oil and Vinegar dressing is allowed, as is Cardini's Original Caesar Salad Dressing. In fact, just about any no-carb, sugar-free dressing will do.

Dairy: In Phase 1, avoid all full-fat ice cream, milk, and yogurt. You can have 1% or fat-free milk, cottage cheese, or fat-free plain yogurt, but no more than two servings a day. You can also use low-fat plain soy milk as a dairy substitute. As for cheese, you can have pretty much any reduced-fat variety. A good rule of thumb is to stick with cheeses containing no more than 6 grams of fat per serving. American cheese slices made with 2% fat milk are fine, as is part-skim ricotta, part-skim mozzarella, or cottage cheese that's made with either 1% or 2% milk fat. Reduced-fat feta cheese is a good choice. But if you can't find reduced-fat feta, the regular kind is ok because it's so flavorful that you don't need to use much.

Eggs: Eggs are allowed even in Phase 1, unless you have dangerously high cholesterol. In truth, eggs aren't nearly as bad as we once thought—they raise the level of the good cholesterol as much as the bad, and they are a terrific source of natural vitamin E. If your doctor has advised you against eating eggs, ask him or her about using an egg substitute.

Fish and shellfish: Fresh halibut, herring, salmon, trout (rainbow or lake), tuna, mackerel, and all other fresh fish are allowed. Smoked salmon, lox, canned salmon, canned tuna, fresh or canned sardines, and smoked whitefish are all okay. Shellfish, such as clams, crab, lobster, shrimp, and so on, are all permitted on the diet. Like meat, fish must be prepared in a healthy way—not breaded and definitely not deep-fried. Fish can be steamed, roasted, grilled, sautéed, and baked. Caviar is high in cholesterol, but a dollop or two is fine now and then.

Flour: Avoid all flour in Phase 1.

Fruit: Avoid all fruit and fruit juices in Phase 1.

Meat and poultry: Most meats are legal. They're a main source of protein, and if you choose carefully, you won't be overdoing the saturated fats. Meat is also good because it satisfies hunger so well. It should always be prepared using healthy methods, though, such as grilling, baking, broiling, roasting, or sautéing—but never frying. When sautéing, use moderate amounts of healthy fats, such as extra virgin olive oil or canola oil, rather than butter or other oils.

In the beef category, sirloin (including ground), tenderloin, top loin, round tip, bottom round, eye round, and top round are all permitted, since they are the leanest cuts. For pork, lean, well-trimmed pork chops or pork tenderloin is acceptable. Boiled ham is okay at this stage, too. Canadian bacon is preferable to its American cousin because it's leaner. Veal chops, cutlets, and top round are legal, as is leg of lamb, well trimmed of fat.

When buying luncheon meats, basically anything fat-free or low-fat is good. Boiled ham is fine, but any ham cured or processed using honey is not. Pastrami, believe it or not, can be acceptable, as long as you can find a lean variety. Low-fat bologna and salami are legal. Sliced turkey breast, turkey hot dogs, and turkey salami are all fine, too.

For poultry, chicken breast, turkey breast, and Cornish game hen are all fine. Dark meat is permitted in limited quantities in Phase 2.

For breakfast meats, Canadian bacon and turkey bacon are fine. Regular bacon is permitted only in moderation because of the saturated fat it contains. The same goes for breakfast sausages—varieties made with turkey (either links or patties) are better than the traditional kind.

If you use meat substitutes, tofu, tempeh, and any other soy-based product is allowed in all phases of the diet. Choose soft, low-fat, or light versions. Soy nuts are permitted. Veggie burgers are also allowed.

Oils: Canola oil, extra virgin olive oil, flaxseed oil, peanut oil, sesame oil, and walnut oil are all fine on all three phases, both for cooking and for salad dressings.

Pasta: No pasta is allowed in Phase 1.

Rice: No rice is allowed in Phase 1.

Snacks: Limit sweet treats to 75 calories per day in Phase 1. Reach for hard, sugar-free candies; unsweetened baking cocoa powder; No-Sugar-Added Fudgsicle Pops; No-Sugar-Added Creamsicle Pops; sugar-free gelatin; and sugar-free gum.

All types of nuts are fine in Phase 1—even macadamias, which we used to think were unhealthy. Almonds are best for the nutrients they contain, but you should really limit consumption of nuts to about 1/4 cup per day.

Soups: Clear broths and reduced-fat canned bean soups are fine in Phase 1.

Sweeteners: You can use any no-calorie sugar substitute you like.

Vegetables: Most vegetables are legal on all phases of the diet. All the green ones can stay. Spinach and the other leafy dark green ones are fine. The same is true for artichokes, asparagus, avocados, beans (black, butter, chickpeas, green, Italian, kidney, lentils, lima, pigeon, soy, split peas, and wax), bell peppers, broccoli, broccoli rabe, cabbage, cauliflower, celery, collard greens, cucumbers, eggplant, fennel, leeks, lettuce (all varieties), mushrooms (all kinds), onions, radishes, scallions, shallots, snow peas, spaghetti squash, sprouts, turnips, water chestnuts, and zucchini. Tomatoes are okay in Phase 1.

Phase 2 Shopping

After the first 2 weeks on the South Beach Diet, you'll enter the Phase 2 eating regimen. In this second phase, you can enjoy all of the foods from Phase 1, plus some additions.

I always advise dieters to reintroduce new carbohydrates gradually—maybe one piece of fruit a day, or a cup of rice or pasta once or twice a week. If it's bread you want, you should be eating true whole grain varieties.

If you add more carbs back to your diet and notice that your weight loss stalls, you've probably gone too far. On the other hand, if you can eat a piece of bread every day without undermining your hard work, feel free.

In Phase 2, you can go out and buy these items:

Baked goods: This is maybe the most confusing aisle in the supermarket. You'll see 7-grain, 9-grain, even 12-grain bread, which might lead you to think you're getting something healthy. But when you read the ingredients, you see that first on the list is enriched white flour—a no-no. You should try to find whole grain bread, which is always available in health food stores. Beyond that, look for bread with 100 percent whole wheat flour as the first ingredient. Or try multigrain, oat and bran, rye, or whole wheat breads. Bread should contain at least 3 grams of dietary fiber per slice. (Pay extra attention here, because some manufacturers will give the information per serving, meaning for two slices.)

There are quite a few flatbreads and crackers made with whole grain wheat that are fine in Phases 2 and 3. Pita bread is also acceptable after the first 2 weeks. Look for stone-ground or whole wheat types. Small, whole grain bagels are fine in Phase 2.

Overall, I suggest no more than one or two starches a day. It can be a slice of whole grain bread with lunch and then a serving of brown rice with dinner. Maybe whole wheat pasta at one meal and mashed sweet potatoes with another. Try to accompany all such carbs with a healthy protein, such as meat, fish, or cheese. Fats will slow down the speed with which your body processes carbs, which is a good thing to do.

When buying breads and baked goods, beware of any hydrogenated oils.

Continue to avoid refined wheat bagels, refined wheat breads, white bread, and dinner rolls.

Beverages: Continue to avoid all fruit juices and sugared sodas in Phase 2. It's okay to have a daily glass or two of red or white wine. It's best to have wine with a meal because your blood sugar will rise less rapidly. But still steer clear of beer. It raises blood sugar much faster than table sugar. Even light beer is out. Whiskey, too, converts to sugar, and should also be avoided, along with all premixed cocktails.

Cereals: Stay away from instant or microwave oatmeal, but feel free to enjoy the old-fashioned kind you cook on the stove. Some cold cereals are fine—Kellogg's All-Bran with Extra Fiber is a good one—but most of them contain too much sugar and too little fiber to be any good for you. Even granola, despite its healthy reputation, usually has too much sugar. You'll see cereal labeled "fat-free," but the fat never was the problem in cereal—it's the bad carbs and sugar.

Avoid cornflakes even in Phase 2.

Condiments, dressings, and seasonings: Barbecue sauce, ketchup, honey mustard, and any other condiment or sauce made with sugar, corn syrup, molasses, or high-fructose corn syrup; fat-free mayonnaise, salad dressings, bottled barbecue sauces, and the like; and sweet pickles and relish are all still off-limits.

Dairy: The same rules as in Phase 1 apply. You can

also add artificially sweetened nonfat flavored yogurt, one 4-ounce serving a day.

Fish and shellfish: It's still a good idea to enjoy lots of fish and shellfish, prepared in healthful ways.

Flour: In Phase 2, you can reintroduce whole wheat flour. Whole wheat flour, buckwheat flour, rye flour, and barley flour are just a few of the many varieties available in supermarkets. There are also flours made from soybeans and chickpeas, which are extremely healthy. There are also many boxed mixes for pancakes, waffles, breads, and so on using these grains instead of enriched white flours. Just make sure no hydrogenated oils are in the mixes.

Fruit: Now it's okay to enjoy fruit. Select apples, apricots, blueberries, cantaloupe, cherries, grapefruit, grapes, kiwifruit, mangoes, oranges, peaches, pears, plums, and strawberries. Even in Phase 2, avoid bananas, canned fruit packed in juice or syrup, pineapple, raisins, watermelon, and all sugared jams.

Meat and poultry: The same meats and poultry you ate in Phase 1 are still great choices in Phase 2. Continue to avoid fatty fowl such as duck and goose and pâté.

Oils: Continue using the same oils in Phase 2 that we used in Phase 1 in limited quantities.

Pasta: If it's made with whole wheat flour, it's approved after Phase 1.

Rice: White rice is forbidden during any phase; you'll be safer eating either basmati rice, brown rice, or wild

Breaking the Rules

You may be surprised to find that a handful of recipes in this book call for small quantities of ingredients that are either "off limits" in a particular phase or "off limits" on the diet in general. Some examples of this are a tablespoon of dry sherry in a Phase 1 beef and pepper salad, a cup of white flour in a Phase 3 quick bread, or 1/2 cup of white sugar in a Phase 3 cheesecake. When we do include these foods, it's because they greatly enhance either the flavor or the texture of a dish, and since the total quantity—which is small to begin with—is spread out over several servings, you don't consume the full amount in your portion.

But just as importantly, these few recipes remind us that a little flexibility goes a long way in adapting the South Beach Diet as a lifestyle. If you stick to the nutritional guidelines of whichever phase you're on, an occasional small detour shouldn't have any lasting effect on your weight loss or overall health goals.

rice (which isn't a rice at all—it's a seed). Steer clear of instant rice.

Snacks: In Phase 2, add chocolate back to your diet sparingly, choosing bittersweet and semi-sweet. Enjoy sugar-free fat-free puddings, too. Air-popped popcorn without oil is a great snack to add in Phase 2. Keep away from the cookies, cupcakes, potato chips, pretzels, and other salty and sweet snacks.

Soup: In Phase 2, you can have canned bean soup, so

long as there's no pasta or other starches included. Powdered soups are always a bad idea—they contain too many carbs.

Sweeteners: After Phase 1, the honey and molasses can come back in moderation, but other sugars should be for special occasions only.

Vegetables: At this point, you may reintroduce sweet potatoes, carrots, and yams to your diet. Continue avoiding beets, corn, and white potatoes. Again, start slowly and monitor what eating these vegetables does to your diet and your cravings.

ASK DR. AGATSTON

As you might imagine, we get lots of questions about foods and methods of preparation. Here are some of the most commonly asked ones.

Is it all right to eat reheated leftovers from dinner for breakfast? I'm not a big fan of eggs.

Leftovers are fine for any meal, as long as they are consistent with the rules for your phase of the diet. It's probably not a great idea to start the day with fruit, pasta, or rice, however. That's because these foods can stimulate cravings for more carbs later. But fish, meat, or vegetables are great choices for breakfast.

Is every kind of bean allowed in all phases of the diet?

Most beans are allowed in all phases, and they're delicious. They're also good sources of nutrients and protein.

Aren't some shellfish—like lobster, for instance—bad for people on a diet or for those of us who have high cholesterol?

No! The amount of cholesterol in shellfish has always been exaggerated because the plant sterols they contain were misunderstood—they are chemically similar to cholesterol, but they actually help decrease cholesterol levels. Lobster has the same amount of cholesterol as skinless chicken breast. All shellfish are low in saturated fat and are not restricted on the diet.

What should I be using instead of butter for cooking and on top of bread or steamed vegetables?

In cooking and on bread, we suggest extra virgin olive oil, which is served with bread at most Mediterranean restaurants. You can add garlic, a little grated cheese, or roasted peppers to the oil for flavor. Atop vegetables, try extra virgin olive oil and lemon instead of butter. We also suggest nonfat cooking sprays. There are also some good vegetable-spread products to use in place of butter, on bread, or anywhere else. Popular brands are Benecol, Take Control, and Smart Balance.

I've tried modified carb diets before but always suffered with constipation as a result. Is there any way to avoid this on the diet?

Yes, there is. You need to maximize your fiber intake by eating plenty of whole grains and whole fruits and vegetables. In all phases, you can also take fiber supplements or psyllium liberally to prevent constipation. Fiber supplements taken with meals actually help control blood sugar and insulin levels and can also help lower your cholesterol.

Is it safe for children to follow the South Beach Diet?

The American epidemic of obesity and diabetes has now extended to our teenagers and pre-teens. The South Beach Diet is the answer to this epidemic, and its principles are exactly the ones that should be applied to our children. The good fats, particularly omega-3 oils, are crucial for the development of young nervous systems, while trans fats are dangerous. The good carbs, including whole grains and whole fruits and vegetables, provide the vitamins, minerals, and nutrients kids especially need. I believe that most children should begin with the Phase 2 eating plan, and you should always consult with your child's pediatrician before putting your child on any diet plan.

Are tomatoes allowed?

Yes, they're fine in all phases, even though technically they are fruits. We even suggest tomato juice or V8 with breakfast. Tomato and tomato sauces contain lycopene, which we think helps prevent prostate cancer.

Which sweeteners are all right for use in cooking and baking?

After Phase 1, applesauce is fine, as long as it has no added sugar. Fruit juices are allowed in cooking, too, but in moderation. You can use a little honey or molasses to impart some of their flavor and moisture, beginning in Phase 2, but you should combine it with a sugar substitute.

Is there any difference between frozen vegetables and fresh?

There's no difference in terms of the diet. In fact, some frozen vegetables have more nutrients than fresh ones because they are blanched and frozen as soon as they're picked, whereas "fresh" produce may sit around on trucks or store shelves for several days before you eat it.

How do I know (other than by weighing myself) if I'm overdoing good carbs once I reintroduce them to my diet? Are there any other signs or symptoms?

The basic guide to success on the South Beach Diet is the disappearance of cravings. This should occur fairly early in Phase 1. If strong cravings for bread, potatoes, and so on recur in Phase 2, you've probably been eating too many carbs, and you need to cut back. Weight loss during Phase 2 should be 1 to 2 pounds per week. If loss has stalled, this is probably the result of too many bad carbs.

Is lamb all right on the diet?

Lamb does contain more saturated fat than beef or chicken, but it's allowed as long as it has been well-trimmed of fat. Roast leg of lamb is best; chops should be a special treat.

I'm a sandwich addict. I also like the convenience of sandwiches. But I don't want to overdo bread by having two slices every day for lunch. Is there an alternative?

It's possible to make sandwiches without bread—take your ingredients, such as turkey, ham, or whatever, add the mustard or mayo, tomato, and seasonings, and wrap it all up in a few leaves of lettuce. You can compromise by using just one slice of whole grain bread or small whole wheat pita.

Are nut butters allowed?

Yes, all are permitted and even encouraged because they're healthy and they taste good. But buy the kind with no added ingredients—natural food stores and even most supermarkets now sell almond, cashew, and peanut butter that consists of the pure nuts with no additional sugars or fats.

Which pickles and relishes are okay?

The sour varieties are fine, but not the sweet. Sugar is added to the vinegar used to make gherkins and other sweet pickles and pickle relish.

Can I have sushi on the diet?

Because of the sticky rice, sushi is for Phase 3 dieters only. But those in Phases 1 and 2 can feel free to eat sashimi, which is sushi without the rice.

What's the difference between whole milk, 2%, 1%, fat-free, and soy, in terms of the diet?

The sugar in dairy takes the form of lactose, which is not harmful to your diet like normal table sugar. But whole milk dairy also contains saturated fat, which is bad for your heart. Because milk is a good source of calcium, you're better off using low-fat or fat free dairy products. Soy milk is a good source of protein and is perfect for people who are lactose-intolerant or just don't like cow's milk. But check the label—some brands add more sugar than others.

Which is better for dessert, frozen yogurt or ice milk?

They're equally bad. There's a lot of sugar in both. Try sugar-free ice pops or fudge pops instead. A small scoop of real ice cream is an okay way to cheat once in a while, and you won't be under the illusion that you've been virtuous. Try mixing it with healthy items such as fruit, or stir in some almonds, peanuts, or walnuts.

Can I make my own sorbet using crushed ice, lemon juice, and sugar substitute?

Sounds perfectly fine—you can't go wrong with those ingredients. But you should probably prepare it and eat it immediately, because with a little time in the freezer, it may turn into a solid rock of lemon ice.

When can I start eating chocolate again, and how should I add it back to my diet?

Even in Phase 1, there's a dessert made using unsweetened cocoa and reduced-fat ricotta cheese that we include in the first book. In Phase 2, you can try having small amounts of dark chocolate, preferably in combination with other things, like strawberries. Try a tiny taste of it to finish off dessert—for example, two or three chocolate espresso beans on top of that cocoa-ricotta dish, or a few squares of really good dark chocolate. (The dark kind has less sugar than milk chocolate.) The key is to keep it under control.

Are olives all right? With pimientos?

They're perfectly fine—olives are as healthy as extra virgin olive oil, a good source of monounsaturated fat. The pimientos are simply peppers, and they are good, too.

Can I have commercial (unsweetened) breakfast cereal with 2% milk?

Not in Phase 1. In Phase 2 you can, but stick with kinds that are highest in fiber and lowest in sugar. Those made with whole grain are best. You should steer clear of cereals made from corn.

Is puff pastry or phyllo dough allowed?

Either one is fairly low in carbs and can be used in cooking and baking in limited amounts, beginning in Phase 2. Typically, you'd brush each layer of phyllo with butter, which *is* a problem. Try it using a butter-flavored cooking spray instead and see if you like it.

I live in the Southwest and love Mexican food. But I know the dishes are high in carbs. Is there a way to get around that?

Sure, if you can resist the taco chips that come as soon as you sit, and then not order a burrito, enchilada, taco, tamale, or tortilla. The rice is also not recommended for dieters on Phases 1 or 2. Try some of the salsa with vegetables instead of chips, and then stick to dishes without any kind of tortilla wrap. Mexican cuisine makes great use of meats and fish in flavorful sauces.

I love salty, packaged snacks, such as corn chips, popcorn, potato chips, pretzels, and the rest. Which of those is worst for dieters?

In terms of the bad carbs, pretzels are worst, followed by corn chips, potato chips, and then packaged popcorn. We've got a terrific recipe for roasted chickpeas (see page 115) that can take the place of these bad items. Air-popped popcorn without butter can be eaten as a snack in Phase 2.

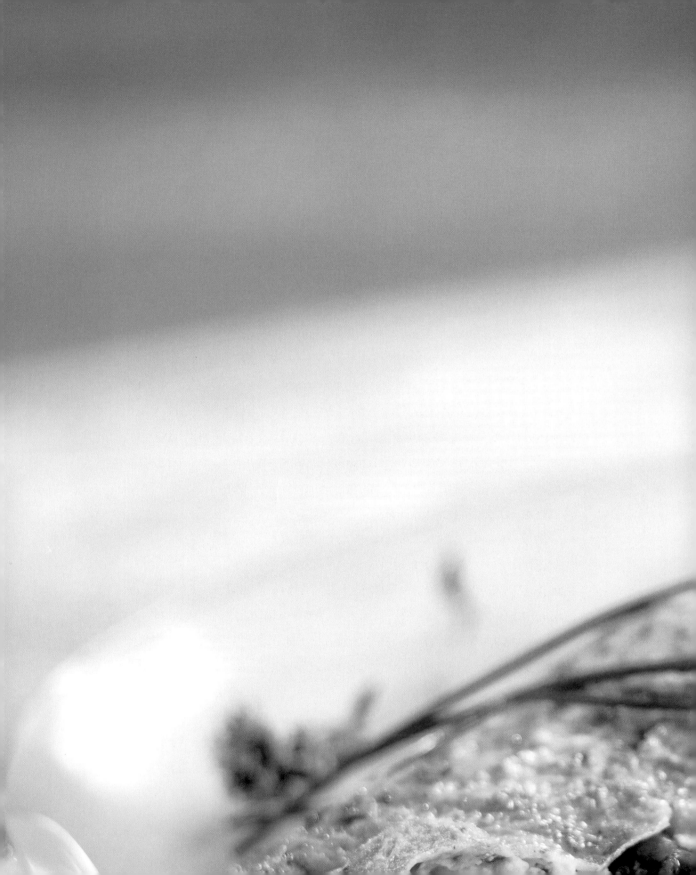

BREAKFASTS

In my medical practice, I've observed that a great many patients who say they never eat breakfast also suffer from obesity. Is there a connection? Quite possibly. Going too long without food can be a problem, because the resulting hunger pangs can cause you to overeat, usually the worst foods. That alone makes it important to start the day with a satisfying meal.

Bad breakfast habits may also set you up for trouble at lunchtime or later. One important study proved that starting the morning with processed carbs—a bagel, say—will stimulate cravings for more of the same throughout the day. The same research has shown that a breakfast of good proteins and fats—like a cheese and vegetable omelet—will actually keep those urges away. Eggs (or egg substitute), vegetables, and lean meats are all healthy ways to start the day.

Oat Smoothie

If you're not a fan of strawberries, you can replace them with the berry of your choice in this quick and delicious breakfast shake.

2 1/2 cups strawberries, halved

1 cup fat-free plain yogurt

1/2 teaspoon sugar substitute

1/4 cup nonfat dry milk

1/4 cup chopped walnuts

3 tablespoons oat bran

2 tablespoons sugar-free pancake syrup

1/2 cup ice cubes

In a blender or food processor, combine the strawberries, yogurt, sugar substitute, dry milk, walnuts, oat bran, syrup, and ice cubes. Blend until smooth and frothy.

Makes 4 servings

NUTRITION AT A GLANCE

Per serving: 130 calories, 6 g fat, 1/2 g saturated fat, 7 g protein, 19 g carbohydrate, 3 g dietary fiber, 0 mg cholesterol, 70 mg sodium

Soy-ous Apricot Muffins

Rather than munching a sugar-full bakery muffin when the urge strikes, enjoy these healthy alternatives as an occasional breakfast on Phase 3. The soy in these muffins provides you with phytochemicals, protein, and dietary fiber and has been proven to reduce "bad" cholesterol.

2	cups whole wheat or whole grain pastry flour
1/4	cup sugar substitute
1/4	cup sugar
1/3	cup soy flour
1	tablespoon baking powder
1	teaspoon ground cinnamon
1/2	teaspoon ground nutmeg
	Pinch of salt
1	egg, beaten
3/4	cup soy milk
3/4	cup unsweetened applesauce
3	tablespoons canola oil
1/3	cup dried apricots, chopped

Preheat the oven to 400°F. Coat a 12-cup nonstick muffin pan with cooking spray or line with paper baking cups.

In a large bowl, thoroughly combine the pastry flour, sugar substitute, sugar, soy flour, baking powder, cinnamon, nutmeg, and salt. Hollow out the center of the dry mixture, and add the egg, soy milk, applesauce, oil, and apricots, stirring until moistened. Pour the batter into the prepared muffin cups.

Bake for 14 minutes, or until a wooden pick inserted into the center of a muffin comes out clean. Allow to cool in the pan for about 10 minutes, then place on a rack to cool completely.

Makes 12 muffins

NUTRITION AT A GLANCE

Per muffin: 140 calories, 5 g fat, 1/2 g saturated fat, 4 g protein, 22 g carbohydrate, 3 g dietary fiber, 20 mg cholesterol, 160 mg sodium

Wholesome Oat Muffins

These healthy muffins are so delicious you'll want to enjoy them for breakfast every day. Make a double batch and freeze half for later.

3/4	cup + 2 tablespoons oats
1	cup buttermilk
1 1/4	cups white whole wheat flour or whole grain flour
1 1/2	teaspoons baking powder
1/2	teaspoon baking soda
1/4	teaspoon ground cinnamon
1/4	teaspoon salt
2/3	cup chopped walnuts
1/3	cup canola oil
1	egg, beaten
1/3	cup brown sugar substitute
1	teaspoon vanilla

Preheat the oven to 425°F. Coat a 12-cup nonstick muffin pan with cooking spray or line with paper baking cups.

In a small bowl, combine 3/4 cup of the oats and the buttermilk. Let soak for 30 minutes.

In a medium bowl, combine the flour, baking powder, baking soda, cinnamon, salt, and walnuts.

In a large bowl, stir together the oil, egg, brown sugar substitute, and vanilla until well blended. Stir in the oat mixture. Stir in the flour mixture until just combined. Do not overmix.

Divide the batter evenly among the prepared muffin cups, filling them about two-thirds full. Sprinkle the remaining 2 tablespoons oats over the muffins. Bake for 11 to 15 minutes, or until a wooden pick inserted in the center of a muffin comes out clean. Cool on a rack for 5 minutes. Remove to the rack to cool completely.

Makes 12 muffins

NUTRITION AT A GLANCE

Per muffin: 180 calories, 10 g fat, 1 g saturated fat, 4 g protein, 21 g carbohydrate, 3 g dietary fiber, 20 mg cholesterol, 191 mg sodium

Apple Walnut Muffins

Chopped fresh apple, not the usual applesauce, flavors these moist muffins. If you really like cinnamon, you can add an extra 1/4 to 1/2 teaspoon for added zip. Make these an occasional part of your Phase 3 breakfast plan.

1 1/2 cups whole wheat or whole grain pastry flour
2 teaspoons baking powder
1 teaspoon baking soda
1 teaspoon ground cinnamon
1/4 teaspoon salt
3/4 cup buttermilk
3 tablespoons canola oil
2 tablespoons packed brown sugar
2 tablespoons sugar substitute
1 egg, beaten
1/2 medium apple, peeled and finely chopped
1/2 cup chopped walnuts

Preheat the oven to 400°F. Coat a 12-cup nonstick muffin pan with cooking spray or line with paper baking cups.

In a medium bowl, combine the flour, baking powder, baking soda, cinnamon, and salt.

In a large bowl, combine the buttermilk, oil, brown sugar, sugar substitute, and egg. Stir in the flour mixture until just combined. Do not overmix. Stir in the apples and walnuts.

Evenly divide the batter among the prepared muffin cups, filling them about two-thirds full. Bake for 12 minutes, or until a wooden pick inserted in the center of a muffin comes out clean. Cool on a rack for 5 minutes. Remove to the rack to cool completely.

Makes 12 muffins

NUTRITION AT A GLANCE

Per muffin: 150 calories, 8 g fat, 1 g saturated fat, 4 g protein, 18 g carbohydrate, 3 g dietary fiber, 20 mg cholesterol, 260 mg sodium

Whole Wheat Loaf

If you have had a difficult time finding a bread at your local grocery store that fits your new diet, perhaps you might want to consider this simple whole wheat bread. It's very easy to make, and the results are just delicious.

1 1/2	cups water (at room temperature)
2 1/2	tablespoons extra virgin olive oil
2	tablespoons sugar substitute
3–3 1/2	cups whole wheat bread flour
2	tablespoons gluten flour
1/2	cup walnuts, chopped
1 1/2	teaspoons salt
1 1/2	teaspoons quick rise yeast

In a large mixing bowl, using an electric mixer, combine the water, oil, sugar substitute, whole wheat bread flour, gluten flour, walnuts, salt, and yeast to form a rough dough. Let the dough stand for 15 to 20 minutes.

Place the dough on a lightly floured board and knead for about 10 minutes, until the dough is smooth and elastic.

Place the dough in an oiled bowl and cover it with a damp cloth. Let the dough rise in a warm spot for about an hour, until it has doubled.

Preheat the oven to 350°F.

Turn the dough onto a board and shape it into an oblong loaf. Coat an 8 1/2" × 4 1/2" bread pan with cooking spray. Place the dough in the pan. Bake the bread for 40 to 45 minutes. Remove the bread from the oven and turn the bread out onto a cooling rack.

Makes 16 slices

NUTRITION AT A GLANCE

Per slice: 130 calories, 5 g fat, 1/2 g saturated fat, 4 g protein, 19 g carbohydrate, 3 g dietary fiber, 0 mg cholesterol, 220 mg sodium

A Guide to Grains and Baked Goods

The biggest adjustment for most people on the South Beach Diet is having to change their relationship with carbohydrates. Many carbs are good for you, and they are an important part of this regimen. Vegetables are carbs, and you'll eat them in abundance. You'll enjoy fruit, too, once you've gotten beyond the first 2 weeks of the program. But to many people, carbs often mean comfy, cozy treats like breads and baked goods.

Some of these carbs—the highly processed packaged ones are going to have to become "once in a great while" treats. There's virtually no way to eat them as often as you once did and still lose weight. Nearly all the fiber and nutrients have been removed in the manufacturing process, leaving only the sugars and starches. They cause you to store excess weight, and they create cravings for even more bad carbs.

But I recognize that a normal diet also will probably include bread, and even muffins or pancakes once in a while. Luckily, you can go on eating these foods while on the South Beach plan. You may even be able to go on using your favorite, traditional recipes for baked goods. It will simply require a little adaptation—replacing the bad grains, which have low fiber, with better ones.

Take bread, for example. The kind that you buy in supermarkets and even in most bakeries is made with all-purpose enriched white flour, from which the whole grain has been removed. Once that grain has been stripped away, the fiber and many of the nutrients go with it. In fact, a useful rule of thumb is that manufacturers use vitamin-enriched flour only when the natural nutrients have been removed during processing. A single slice of white bread contains the equivalent impact on your blood sugar of a tablespoon of pure white sugar, straight from the bowl. Many people eat that bread with breakfast, lunch, and dinner. You can imagine the effect of six or more slices a day on your attempts to lose weight.

If you take any recipe and replace at least some of the white flour with whole wheat flour, or rye or soy flour, you increase the amount of fiber and decrease the degree to which it raises your blood sugar level. You still won't be able to consume six slices a day, but bread will be back on your eating plan without wrecking your diet. The same is true for muffins and pancakes.

You can usually find several kinds of flour in the supermarket, nearly all of which are better for you than the traditional bleached white, all-purpose kind. Here's how to get bread and baked goods back into your diet, once you've reached Phase 3. In Phase 2, you should still try to avoid white flour.

Bread: You can take any recipe for white bread and replace half the flour with whole wheat flour. It's that simple. You can also try rye flour, which comes in three varieties: light, medium, and dark. Rye flour imparts an interesting, slightly sour flavor to bread. Because rye flour is denser than white flour, you should increase the amount of yeast so that the bread rises properly. If you use light rye flour, replace half the white flour with it. If using medium rye flour, replace one-third of the white flour. If using dark rye flour, replace no more than one-quarter of the white flour in your bread recipe. There's even something called dark rye meal, which will give you pumpernickel bread—dark, dense, and very tasty.

You can also make bread using buckwheat flour or oat flour. Replace one-quarter of the white flour with the oat flour, and increase the yeast slightly, too.

"Quick breads" and muffins: "Quick bread" means any kind made using baking powder and baking soda instead of yeast. The dough doesn't rise—you just bake the batter. You can simply replace half the white flour with whole wheat. Whole wheat flour is coarser than white flour, so do not try to sift it. Quick breads made with whole wheat flour will have a nutty flavor and may have slightly less volume than those made with white flour.

You can make muffins with oat bran instead of flour, too. You can also use barley flour, which has a mild taste, or oat flour, which is especially good in cookies.

Pancakes: You can readily find pancake mixes made with buckwheat. The taste may take a little getting used to, but they're quite good served with sugar-free maple syrup and one of the heart-healthy (trans-free) butter substitutes. Or if you're making pancakes from scratch, replace up to one-fifth of the white flour in your favorite pancake recipe with buckwheat flour.

You can also make homemade pancakes using whole wheat flour. Even oat bran can be used to make terrific pancakes.

Breakfast Popovers with Parmesan

Here's a popover that's sure to please. For variety, you can swap the Parmesan for other cheeses, such as freshly grated Romano or Asiago cheese.

1/2	cup liquid egg substitute
1 1/4	cups whole grain flour
1	cup + 2 tablespoons fat-free milk
1	tablespoon trans-free margarine, melted
3	tablespoons grated Parmesan cheese

Preheat the oven to 375°F. Coat 8 custard cups or popover-pan cups with cooking spray.

Whisk the egg substitute in a medium bowl. Add the flour, milk, and margarine, and whisk until the ingredients are combined. Stir in the cheese.

Evenly divide the batter among the prepared cups. Place the cups on a large baking sheet.

Bake for 30 minutes, or until the popovers are puffed and golden. Remove the popovers from the cups and serve hot.

Makes 8 popovers

NUTRITION AT A GLANCE

Per popover: 110 calories, 2 1/2 g fat, 1/2 g saturated fat, 6 g protein, 15 g carbohydrate, 2 1/2 g dietary fiber, 0 mg cholesterol, 95 mg sodium

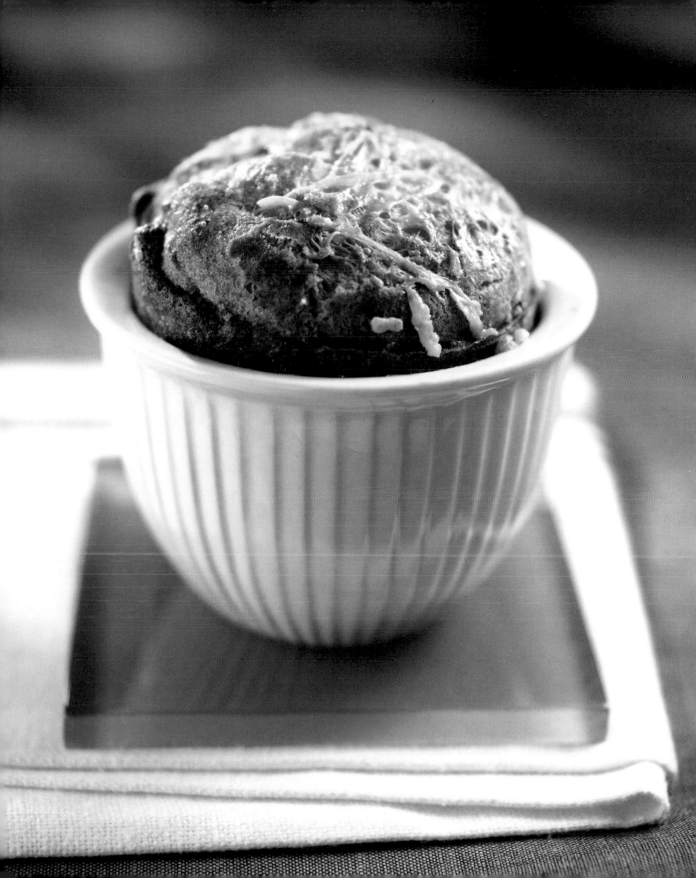

Quick Nut Bread

This is called a quick bread because it is made without yeast. You can easily alter this recipe to include your favorite flavor with a couple of simple ingredient changes. This bread may be baked in virtually anything that you can put in your oven; just remember to fill the container only three-quarters full. If you don't, it will overflow when it expands, and you'll have a big mess to clean up!

1/3	cup sugar substitute
1/3	cup sugar
1/3	cup canola oil
1	egg, beaten
1 1/2	cups fat-free milk
1 1/2	cups all-purpose flour
1	cup whole wheat flour
1	tablespoon baking powder
1/2	teaspoon baking soda
1	teaspoon salt
1	cup finely chopped walnuts

Preheat the oven to 350°F. Coat a 9" × 5" loaf pan with cooking spray.

In a medium bowl, thoroughly combine the sugar substitute, sugar, oil, and egg. Stir in the milk. Add the all-purpose flour, whole wheat flour, baking powder, baking soda, and salt, and stir until smooth. Fold in the nuts. Place the mixture into the prepared pan.

Bake for 1 hour, or until the loaf is brown on the top and firm to the touch in the center. Cool in the pan for 15 minutes, then remove from the pan and cool on a rack. For easiest slicing, refrigerate to cool further before slicing.

Makes 1 loaf

NUTRITION AT A GLANCE

Per slice: 200 calories, 10 g fat, 1 g saturated fat, 5 g protein, 24 g carbohydrate, 2 g dietary fiber, 15 mg cholesterol, 290 mg sodium

Pancakes with Peachy Compote

This delicious combination will fast become a breakfast favorite.

Compote

    1 peach, sliced, or 1 cup drained sliced canned peaches (not in syrup)
  1/4 cup orange juice
    3 tablespoons sugar-free apricot preserves
    1 teaspoon finely chopped crystallized ginger
  1/2 teaspoon ground cinnamon
    2 cups blackberries or blueberries

Pancakes

    2 cups whole wheat or whole grain pastry flour
    1 teaspoon baking soda
  1/2 teaspoon baking powder
  1/2 teaspoon salt
    1 egg
    1 egg white
    2 cups buttermilk
    1 tablespoon vanilla extract
    2 teaspoons canola oil

To make the compote: In a small saucepan, combine the peaches, orange juice, preserves, ginger, and cinnamon. Cook, stirring occasionally, over medium heat for 5 minutes, or until the fruit is soft. Add the berries and cook for 2 minutes longer. Keep warm over very low heat.

To make the pancakes: In a large bowl, combine the flour, baking soda, baking powder, and salt.

In a medium bowl, whisk together the egg and egg white until very foamy. Whisk in the buttermilk, vanilla extract, and oil. Stir into the flour mixture just until the batter is combined and pourable.

Heat a large nonstick skillet coated with cooking spray over medium heat. Pour 1/3 cup batter into the skillet to form a 4" pancake. Cook for 2 to 3 minutes, or until the bottom is browned. Turn and cook for 1 to 2 minutes longer, or until golden brown. Remove to a plate and keep warm. Repeat to make a total of 12 pancakes. Serve the pancakes with the warm compote.

Makes 12 pancakes

NUTRITION AT A GLANCE

Per pancake: 130 calories, 2 g fat, 0 g saturated fat, 5 g protein, 24 g carbohydrate, 3 g dietary fiber, 20 mg cholesterol, 280 mg sodium

Buckwheat Pancakes

Buckwheat sounds like a grain, but it is really a summer annual. It is often planted by beekeepers, because the flower is very high in nectar. The popularity of the buckwheat pancake has declined since the 1950s, but there's no reason not to try them today!

- 1 cup buckwheat flour
- 1 cup whole wheat flour
- 1 egg, beaten
- 1 tablespoon baking powder
- 2 cups water
- 1/2 cup unsweetened applesauce
- 1 teaspoon vanilla extract

In a medium bowl, thoroughly combine the buckwheat flour, whole wheat flour, egg, and baking powder, mixing until evenly blended. Add the water, applesauce, and vanilla extract, and stir until only small lumps remain.

Heat a large nonstick skillet coated with cooking spray over medium heat. Working in batches, pour the batter into the pan and cook for 2 to 3 minutes, or until the bottom is browned. Turn and cook for 1 to 2 minutes longer, or until golden brown. Remove to a plate and keep warm. Repeat to make a total of 12 pancakes.

Makes 12 pancakes

NUTRITION AT A GLANCE

Per pancake: 80 calories, 1 g fat, 0 g saturated fat, 3 g protein, 16 g carbohydrate, 2 g dietary fiber, 20 mg cholesterol, 130 mg sodium

Oatmeal Pancakes

These tend to be somewhat dense pancakes. If you would like to change the flavor, all you need to do is add cinnamon, nutmeg, cloves, or a teaspoon of your favorite extract flavoring.

1 1/4 cups rolled oats

2 cups fat-free milk

1 egg

1/2 cup whole wheat flour

1/4 cup toasted wheat germ

1 tablespoon baking powder

2 teaspoons sugar substitute

2 teaspoons canola oil

1/2 teaspoon salt

In a medium bowl, combine the oats and milk and allow to stand for 10 minutes. Stir in the egg, flour, wheat germ, baking powder, sugar substitute, oil, and salt, mixing until evenly blended and only small lumps remain. Let the batter stand for 30 minutes in the refrigerator.

Heat a large nonstick skillet coated with cooking spray over medium heat. Working in batches, pour the batter by 1/4 cup into the pan and cook for 3 to 4 minutes, or until the top starts to bubble and the bottom is browned. Turn and cook for 1 to

2 minutes longer, or until golden brown. Remove to a plate and keep warm. Repeat to make a total of 12 pancakes.

Makes 12 pancakes

NUTRITION AT A GLANCE

Per pancake: 90 calories, 2 g fat, 0 g saturated fat, 1/2 g protein, 14 g carbohydrate, 1 g dietary fiber, 20 mg cholesterol, 250 mg sodium

Cottage Cheese Crêpes with Cherries

Kamut's appealing, nutty flavor lends itself quite nicely to these crêpes.

Crêpes

- 1/3 cup kamut flour
- 2 tablespoons whole wheat or whole grain pastry flour
- 1/8 teaspoon salt
- 1/3 cup apple juice
- 1/2 cup + 1–2 tablespoons water
- 1 large egg, lightly beaten
- 4 teaspoons trans-free margarine

Filling

- 1 cup reduced-fat cottage cheese or reduced-fat ricotta cheese, at room temperature
- 2 cups pitted sweet cherries
- 1/4 cup sugar-free maple syrup

To make the crêpes: In a large bowl, combine the kamut flour, pastry flour, and salt. In a small bowl, whisk together the apple juice, 1/2 cup water, egg, and 2 teaspoons of the margarine. Whisk into the flour mixture to make a smooth batter. Melt 1 teaspoon of the remaining margarine in an 8" nonstick skillet coated with cooking spray over medium heat. Pour 3 tablespoons of batter into the skillet and tilt the skillet to coat the bottom with a thin layer of the batter. (If the

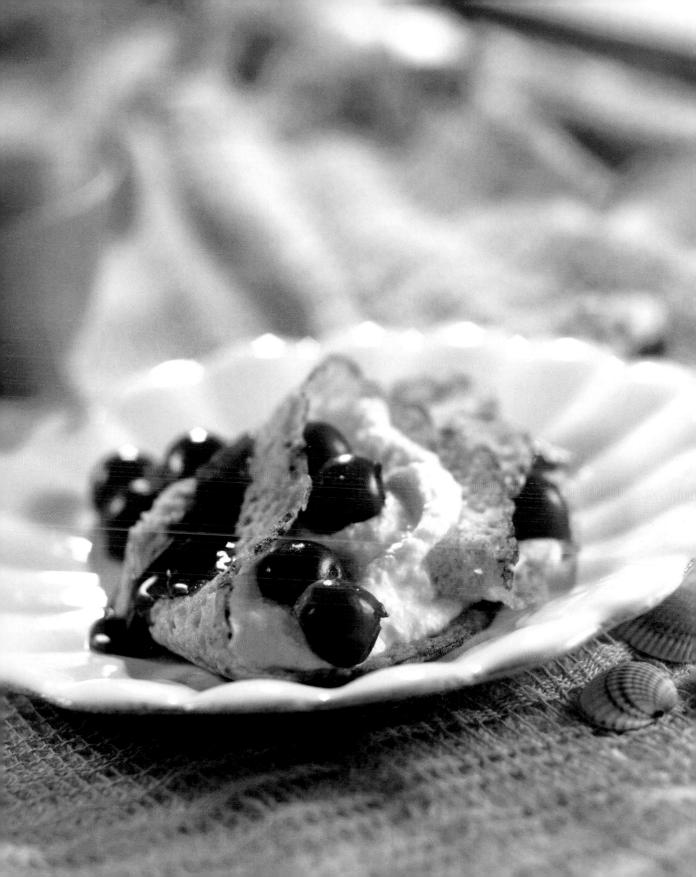

batter seems too thick, add 1 to 2 tablespoons water.) Cook the first side for 1 minute, or until lightly browned. Turn and cook the second side for 30 to 60 seconds. Slide the crepe onto a plate. Cover with foil to keep warm. Continue making crêpes in the same fashion, adding the last teaspoon of margarine to the pan after making the second crêpe.

To make the filling and assemble: Place a crêpe on a plate, attractive side down. Arrange 1/4 cup of the cheese and 1/2 cup of the cherries in a line in the center of the crêpe and fold in quarters. Repeat with the remaining ingredients to make 4 crêpes. Drizzle with syrup.

Makes 4 crêpes

NUTRITION AT A GLANCE

Per crêpe: 220 calories, 7 g fat, 1 1/2 g saturated fat, 13 g protein, 32 g carbohydrate, 4 g dietary fiber, 60 mg cholesterol, 400 mg sodium

MY SOUTH BEACH DIET

WE COULD EAT THIS WAY FOR THE REST OF OUR LIVES.

Our only daughter left for college last year, and my husband, Jack, and I were dealing with "empty nest" feelings, not to mention the added stress of turning 50! Major turning points like these get you thinking about the future. We both gained weight in our forties, and have family histories of heart disease. When the cardiologist said that Jack's high cholesterol readings should be a wake-up call, we knew we had to get serious about making changes.

I picked up the South Beach Diet book after hearing about it in *Prevention* magazine. What really caught my attention was the clear description of the connections between cholesterol, diet, and heart health.

We decided that we were ready to tackle this new preventive lifestyle change together. Jack has always been a morning-coffee-and-pastry guy, not a big egg eater, so finding breakfasts that he enjoyed was tough those first weeks. Learning the basic foods to avoid from the start was really helpful. When I missed my potatoes, I tried Surprise South Beach Mashed "Potatoes," made with cauliflower, and loved them!

After the first 2 weeks (Phase 1), my husband dropped 8 pounds, and I lost 6. It wasn't as much as we'd hoped, but we both had much more energy in the summer evenings for walks or even a round of golf after work. We planned our meals together and found ourselves eating out less. When we do go out, we've been choosing restaurants that serve Mediterranean food—hummus, couscous, grilled fish, meats, and vegetables. Or we focus on trying new salads, and choose main dishes to share.

Jack struggled to stay on the plan while traveling for work—that was probably the hardest challenge so far. Funny coincidence, he sat next to a woman on a plane who shared that it was the first time she didn't need a seatbelt extender, thanks to a new diet. Turns out she'd been on the South Beach Diet, too!

Early success really convinced us to stay with the plan. Jack is now down 15 pounds, and I've lost 12. Jack's cholesterol follow-up is next month, and we're anticipating an improvement. The boost in energy and minimal cravings for old familiar foods made it clear that we could eat this way for the rest of our lives. We can't wait to see our daughter's face when she returns home for the holidays!

—*CYNTHIA AND JACK C.*

Asparagus Omelets with Goat Cheese

The goat cheese gives these omelets a unique savory creaminess.

> 1 cup liquid egg substitute
>
> 4 eggs
>
> 1/4 cup fat-free milk
>
> 2 tablespoons chopped scallions
>
> 2 tablespoons chopped fresh thyme leaves
>
> 2 tablespoons chopped parsley
>
> 1/2 teaspoon ground black pepper
>
> 1/8 teaspoon salt
>
> 1/2 pound asparagus, trimmed and cut into 1" pieces
>
> 1/4 cup water
>
> 4 tablespoons crumbled reduced-fat goat cheese
>
> Chives, for garnish

In a medium bowl, whisk together the egg substitute, eggs, and milk. Stir in the scallions, thyme, parsley, pepper, and salt.

Place the asparagus and water in a large microwaveable bowl. Cover with vented plastic wrap and microwave on high power for 4 minutes, or until crisp-tender. Stop and stir after 2 minutes. Drain, pat dry, and add to the egg mixture.

Heat a medium nonstick skillet coated with cooking spray over medium heat. Pour one-quarter of the egg

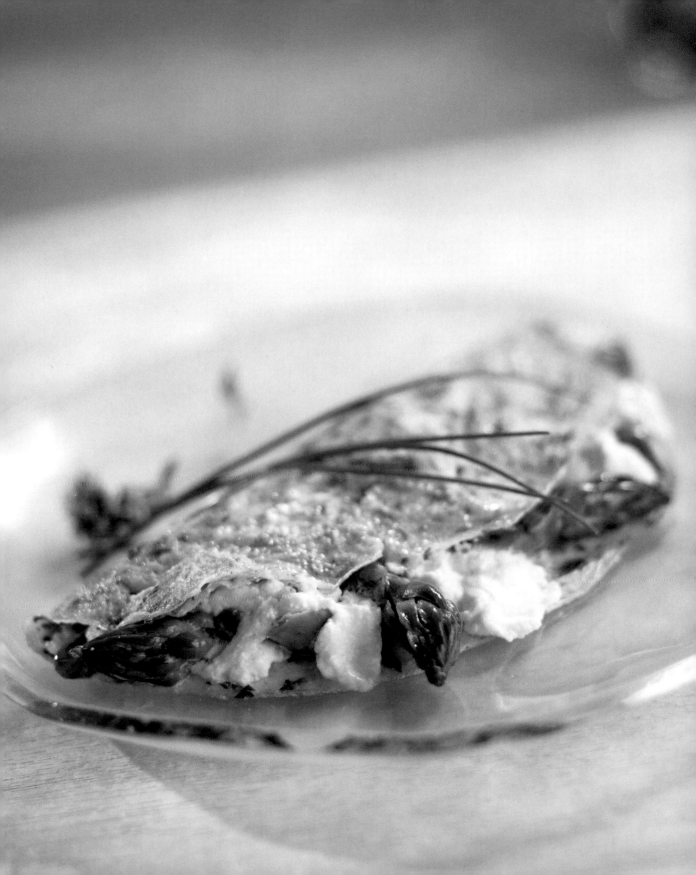

mixture into the skillet, allowing it to cover the bottom of the pan. Cook for 2 to 3 minutes, or until the bottom just begins to set. Sprinkle with 1 tablespoon of the cheese. Add one-quarter of the asparagus pieces. Cook for 5 minutes, or until the eggs are almost set.

Using a large spatula, fold the omelet in half. Cook for 3 minutes, or until the omelet is golden and the cheese is melted. Turn onto a plate and keep warm.

Coat the skillet with cooking spray and repeat the process with the remaining ingredients to make 3 more omelets. Garnish with the chives.

Makes 4 omelets

NUTRITION AT A GLANCE
Per omelet: 180 calories, 9 g fat, 3 g saturated fat, 19 g protein, 6 g carbohydrate, 2 g dietary fiber, 215 mg cholesterol, 450 mg sodium

Vegetable Frittata with Parmesan

This hearty frittata is chock-full of healthy veggies, making for a very satisfying Phase 1 breakfast.

2	tablespoons trans-free margarine
1	onion, chopped
2	zucchini, thinly sliced
4	large mushrooms, chopped
1/2	large red bell pepper, chopped
1/2	teaspoon salt
1/4	teaspoon dried thyme, crushed
1/4	teaspoon ground black pepper
4	large eggs, at room temperature
1	cup liquid egg substitute
1 1/2	tablespoons grated Parmesan cheese (optional)

Place the broiler rack in the lowest position (6 to 7" from the heat source) and preheat the broiler.

Melt 1 tablespoon of the margarine in a large oven-safe nonstick skillet over medium heat. Add the onion, zucchini, mushrooms, bell pepper, 1/4 teaspoon of the salt, the thyme, and 1/8 teaspoon of the pepper. Cook, stirring occasionally, for 8 minutes, or until the vegetables are tender and no juices remain in the pan.

In a large bowl, combine the eggs, egg substitute, the remaining 1/4 teaspoon salt, the remaining 1/8 teaspoon pepper, and the cheese, if using.

Melt the remaining 1 tablespoon margarine in the skillet with the vegetables over very low heat. Pour in the egg mixture. Cook, uncovered and without stirring, for 15 minutes, or until only the top remains runny. Place the skillet under the broiler and cook for 2 minutes, or until the eggs are just set. Slide the frittata onto a large serving plate to serve.

Makes 4 servings

NUTRITION AT A GLANCE

Per serving: 200 calories, 12 g fat, 3 1/2 g saturated fat, 16 g protein, 9 g carbohydrate, 2 g dietary fiber, 215 mg cholesterol, 510 mg sodium

Smoked Ham "Soufflé"

This mock soufflé is healthier than many other breakfast foods and easier to make, too. You can assemble it in the morning and bake it later when you're ready.

　　2　eggs
　　4　egg whites
　1 1/2　cups fat-free milk
　1 1/2　cups (6 ounces) shredded reduced-fat extra-sharp
　　　　Cheddar cheese
　　4　slices light whole wheat bread, cubed
　　1　can (4 ounces) sliced mushrooms, drained
　　1　cup broccoli florets or 2 spears asparagus, trimmed
　　　　and chopped
　　4　ounces lean smoked ham, chopped
　1/2　teaspoon dried Italian seasoning

Preheat the oven to 350°F. Coat a 2-quart baking dish with cooking spray.

In a large bowl, beat the eggs and egg whites until frothy. Stir in the milk, cheese, bread, mushrooms, broccoli or asparagus, ham, and Italian seasoning. Pour into the prepared baking dish.

Bake for 45 minutes, or until golden and a knife inserted in the center comes out clean.

Makes 4 servings

NUTRITION AT A GLANCE

Per serving: 310 calories, 13 g fat, 7 g saturated fat, 29 g protein, 18 g carbohydrate, 3 g dietary fiber, 145 mg cholesterol, 1,080 mg sodium

Sausage and Cheese Breakfast Cups

These egg "muffins" make a hearty breakfast that can be eaten on the run. Make them ahead and warm them in the microwave for a fast and slimming breakfast treat.

4	ounces turkey sausage or crumbled turkey bacon
1/2	green bell pepper, chopped
1/4	onion, chopped
5	large eggs
1	can (12 ounces) sliced mushrooms, drained
1/2	cup (2 ounces) shredded reduced-fat Cheddar cheese

Preheat the oven to 350°F. Coat a 6-cup nonstick muffin pan with cooking spray or line with paper baking cups.

In a medium nonstick skillet over medium-high heat, cook the sausage, pepper, and onion for 5 minutes, or until the sausage is no longer pink. Spoon the mixture into a bowl and cool slightly. Stir in the eggs and mushrooms. Evenly divide the mixture among the prepared muffin cups. Sprinkle with the cheese.

Bake for 20 minutes, or until the egg is set.

Makes 6 cups

NUTRITION AT A GLANCE

Per serving: 140 calories, 9 g fat, 3 g saturated fat, 12 g protein, 4 g carbohydrate, 1 g dietary fiber, 195 mg cholesterol, 400 mg sodium

Quiche with Swiss and Fennel

*The distinct personalities of fennel and Swiss are made for
each other in this South Beach version of a French classic.
Enjoy this dish for breakfast or brunch, or impress company
by serving it as an hors d'oeuvre at your next get-together.*

Crust

1 1/4	cups whole wheat or whole grain pastry flour
1/4	teaspoon salt
2	tablespoons canola oil
2	tablespoons trans-free margarine, cold and cut into small pieces
2–3	tablespoons ice water

Filling

1	cup thinly sliced fennel bulb
6	medium scallions, chopped
4	eggs
1	cup fat-free evaporated milk
1/2	cup fat-free milk
1 1/2	teaspoons Dijon mustard
1/4	teaspoon ground nutmeg
1/4	teaspoon ground black pepper
1/2	cup (2 ounces) shredded reduced-fat Swiss cheese
1	tablespoon grated Parmesan cheese
	Pinch of paprika
	Fennel frond, for garnish

To make the crust: Preheat the oven to 425°F. Coat a 9" pie plate with cooking spray.

In a large bowl or food processor, combine the flour and salt. Blend with a pastry blender or process briefly to mix. Add the oil and margarine and stir or process until the mixture resembles fine meal. While stirring constantly or with the motor of the food processor running, add the water, 1 tablespoon at a time, and stir or process for 30 seconds, or until the dough barely comes together. Remove to a counter and pat the dough into a flattened disk.

Place the dough between 2 sheets of waxed paper and roll out to an 11" circle. Remove the top sheet and invert the dough into the prepared pie plate. Remove

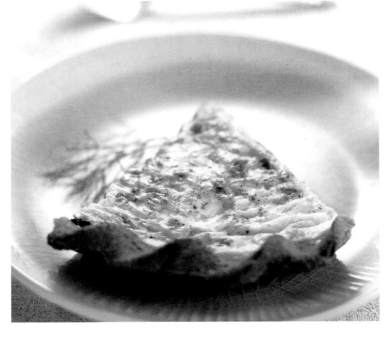

the remaining sheet of waxed paper and fit the dough into the plate. Use a fork to poke holes in the bottom and sides of the dough. Line the dough with a piece of foil and top it with a layer of pie weights or dried rice or beans.

Bake for 10 minutes. Remove the weights and foil and bake for 4 minutes longer, or until the dough is dry but has not begun to brown.

To make the filling: Heat a medium nonstick skillet coated with cooking spray over medium heat. Add the fennel bulb and cook for 5 minutes, or until soft. Add the scallions and cook for 2 minutes.

In a medium bowl, whisk together the eggs, evaporated milk, fat-free milk, mustard, nutmeg, and pepper.

Sprinkle the fennel mixture over the bottom of the baked pie shell and top with the Swiss. Pour in the egg mixture and sprinkle the top with the Parmesan and paprika.

Bake for 30 minutes, or until a knife inserted in the center comes out clean. Cool on a rack for 10 minutes. Garnish with the fennel frond.

Makes 6 servings

NUTRITION AT A GLANCE

Per serving: 280 calories, 14 g fat, 4 g saturated fat, 13 g protein, 27 g carbohydrate, 4 g dietary fiber, 150 mg cholesterol, 290 mg sodium

Hot Scrambled Tofu

Between the hot-pepper sauce and the hot-pepper cheese, this meal is sure to warm you up.

> 2 boxes (10 ounces each) silken tofu
>
> 2 tablespoons extra virgin olive oil
>
> 4 scallions, white part only, minced
>
> 1/4 tablespoon ground turmeric
>
> Salt
>
> Freshly ground black pepper
>
> Hot-pepper sauce
>
> 1/2 cup grated reduced-fat hot-pepper cheese
>
> 1/4 teaspoon paprika

Cover a large baking sheet with paper towels. Place the tofu on the towels in a single layer. Cover the tofu with paper towels and pat down until dry. Discard all of the paper towels. Crumble the tofu.

Heat the oil in a large skillet over medium–high heat. Add the scallions and cook, stirring frequently, for 3 minutes, or until soft. Stir in the tofu and turmeric. Add the salt, pepper, and pepper sauce to taste. Cook for 2 minutes, or until the tofu is firm.

Evenly divide among 4 serving plates. Sprinkle with the cheese and paprika.

Makes 4 servings

NUTRITION AT A GLANCE

Per serving: 190 calories, 14 g fat, 3 1/2 g saturated fat, 11 g protein, 6 g carbohydrate, 7 g dietary fiber, 10 mg cholesterol, 135 mg sodium

Breakfast Croque Monsieur

Why not have this classic ham and cheese sandwich for breakfast? This is good for Phases 2 or 3.

8 slices light whole wheat bread, crusts removed

1/4 cup trans-free margarine, melted

4 ounces reduced-fat mozzarella cheese, thinly sliced

6 ounces boiled ham, thinly sliced

Brush 1 side of each slice of bread with the margarine. Place cheese slices on the side of the bread with the margarine. Add the ham and cover with the remaining bread, dry side up.

Generously brush a large unheated skillet with margarine. Working in batches if necessary, add the sandwiches and cook over medium heat for 4 minutes, or until lightly browned on the bottom. Turn the sandwiches over and rebrush the skillet with margarine. Cover and cook for 4 minutes, or until the cheese is melted and the bread is browned. Serve immediately.

Makes 4 sandwiches

NUTRITION AT A GLANCE

Per sandwich: 280 calories, 16 g fat, 6 g saturated fat, 20 g protein, 20 g carbohydrate, 3 g dietary fiber, 35 mg cholesterol, 1,050 mg sodium

Turkey Patties with Fennel

Fennel seeds lend zip to these tasty sausage patties. If you like, you can substitute 2 tablespoons whole wheat bread crumbs for the chopped nuts to make this a Phase 2 recipe.

1	pound 99% fat-free ground turkey breast
1/4	onion, grated
1	egg, beaten
2	tablespoons finely chopped pecans
1/4	teaspoon fennel seeds, finely crushed

In a bowl, combine the turkey, onion, egg, pecans, and fennel. Shape the turkey mixture into 8 patties.

Heat a large nonstick skillet coated with cooking spray over medium heat for 1 minute. Working in batches if necessary, add the patties and cook for 5 minutes on each side, or until a thermometer inserted in the center of a patty registers 165°F and the meat is no longer pink.

Makes 8 patties

NUTRITION AT A GLANCE

Per patty: 80 calories, 2 g fat, 0 g saturated fat, 15 g protein, 1 g carbohydrate, 0 g dietary fiber, 50 mg cholesterol, 40 mg sodium

Grilled Canadian Bacon

Ten minutes is all it takes to make this crispy bacon. Feel free to use any sugar-free preserve you'd like.

> 1 pound Canadian bacon, cut into 1/4" slices
> 1/4 cup sugar-free apricot preserves
> 1/4 teaspoon mustard powder

Preheat the broiler.

Place the bacon on a broiler rack 3" from the heat and cook for 4 minutes.

In a small bowl, combine the preserves and mustard. Turn the bacon and brush with the preserve mixture. Broil for 4 minutes longer, or until the bacon is well-done.

Makes 4 servings

NUTRITION AT A GLANCE

Per serving: 150 calories, 6 g fat, 2 g saturated fat, 19 g protein, 7 g carbohydrate, 0 g dietary fiber, 55 mg cholesterol, 1,150 mg sodium

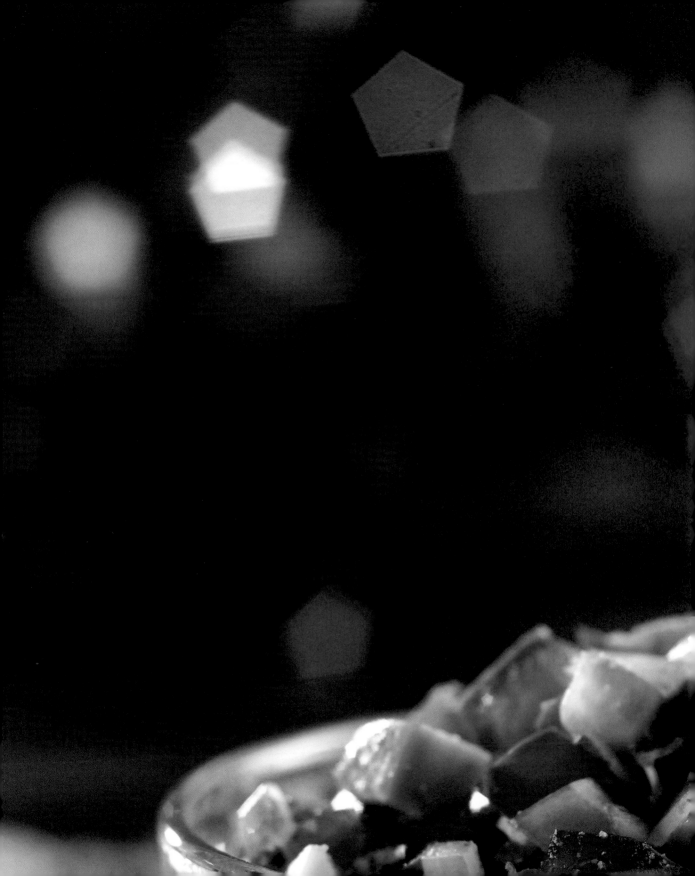

APPETIZERS AND SNACKS

These little tidbits are an extremely important component of the South Beach Diet. Two of the most dangerous times in a dieter's day are the hours between breakfast and lunch—that 10:30 or so coffee break with a bagel, doughnut, or something similar—and then that point in mid-afternoon when your energy begins to flag, and you reach for a pick-me-up of caffeine and sugar, in the form of a candy bar or some kind of baked item. Nothing undermines self-control like the combination of hunger and weariness, and next thing you know, you've acquired an unwanted new habit, one that can undo all your good efforts the rest of the day. This is why we decided that this eating plan would allow you at least two snacks daily.

As you'll see, these dishes are healthy, but they will satisfy your between-meal cravings without filling you with bad carbs. You'll make them again and again.

Lettuce Wrappers with Shrimp

This impressive appetizer wraps hot-and-spicy shrimp in cool-and-crisp lettuce. Save any leftovers for a light yet satisfying lunch the next day.

- 1 tablespoon peanut oil
- 1 pound large shrimp, peeled, deveined, and coarsely chopped
- 1/2 cup finely chopped celery
- 1/4 cup water chestnuts, chopped
- 1 clove garlic, minced
- 1 teaspoon finely chopped fresh ginger
- 1 tablespoon hoisin sauce
- 1 tablespoon light soy sauce
- 1 tablespoon rice wine vinegar
- 8 large leaves Boston lettuce
- Toasted chopped peanuts

Heat the oil in a wok or large nonstick skillet over medium-high heat. Add the shrimp and stir-fry until they are opaque. Remove the shrimp to a bowl and set aside.

Add the celery, water chestnuts, garlic, and ginger, and stir-fry until the vegetables are crisp-tender.

Return the shrimp to the wok and add the hoisin sauce, soy sauce, and vinegar. Cook for 1 minute, or until heated through.

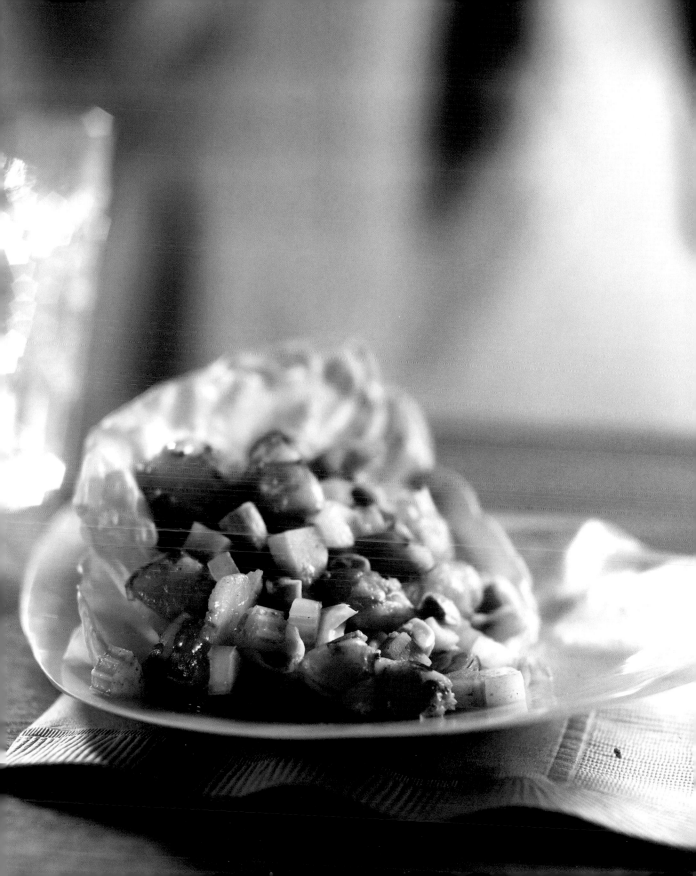

Evenly divide the shrimp mixture among the lettuce leaves. Garnish with the peanuts.

Makes 4 servings

NUTRITION AT A GLANCE

Per serving: 80 calories, 6 g fat, 1 g saturated fat, 2 g protein, 6 g carbohydrate, 2 g dietary fiber, 0 mg cholesterol, 210 mg sodium

Asian Grilled Tempeh Triangles

Tempeh is a soy-based protein that's frequently enjoyed by vegetarians as a meat alternative. You can serve these triangles as an appetizer or with steamed or stir-fried vegetables as a main dish.

- 1 pound soy tempeh, cut into triangles
- 1 tablespoon peanut oil
- 1/2 teaspoon toasted sesame oil
- 1 teaspoon grated ginger
- 2 tablespoons light soy sauce
- 1 teaspoon minced garlic
- 2 tablespoons sliced scallions, for garnish

Place the tempeh in a glass pie plate or dish. In a small bowl mix, the peanut oil, sesame oil, ginger, soy sauce, and garlic. Pour the mixture over the tempeh, turning the pieces to coat well. Place in the refrigerator for 4 hours or overnight.

Heat the grill to medium high heat. Lay a large piece of foil on the grill. Place the tempeh triangles on the foil and grill them for 3 to 4 minutes per side, until golden brown. Sprinkle the tempeh with scallions.

Makes 4 servings

NUTRITION AT A GLANCE

Per serving: 242 calories, 14 g fat, 3 g saturated fat, 22 g protein, 11 g carbohydrate, 7 g dietary fiber, 0 mg cholesterol, 313 mg sodium

From the Menu of . . .
PASHA'S
900 Lincoln Road, Miami Beach

CHEFS TULIN TUZEL AND CARLA ELLEK

PASHA'S SERVES HEALTHY AND DELICIOUS MEDITERRANEAN FOOD, PROVING ONCE AGAIN THE TWO ARE NEVER MUTUALLY EXCLUSIVE.

Artichokes in Olive Oil
PHASE 1

4 globe artichokes, trimmed down to the hearts, retaining part of the stalk

8 scallions, cut into 1" pieces

1 medium onion, sliced

4 teaspoons extra virgin olive oil

1 lemon, sliced

Juice of 1 lemon

1/2 cup water

2 teaspoons salt

6 tablespoons fresh dill

Lemon wedges, for garnish

Place the artichokes in a pan with the scallions, onion, oil, lemon, lemon juice, and water. Cover and cook over low heat for 35 minutes.

Add the salt and most of the dill, reserving some dill for garnish. Baste the artichokes and continue to cook for 20 minutes, or until tender.

Allow the mixture to cool, then garnish with the remaining dill. Serve cold with wedges of lemon for garnish.

Makes 4 servings

NUTRITION AT A GLANCE

Per serving: 110 calories, 5 g fat, 1/2 g saturated fat, 4 g protein, 15 g carbohydrate, 5 g dietary fiber, 0 mg cholesterol, 200 mg sodium

Grilled Clams Gremolata

The word gremolata *means a mixture of minced parsley, garlic, and lemon peel. It adds a fresh, light flavor when sprinkled over seafood.*

> 3 tablespoons chopped parsley
>
> 2 cloves garlic, minced
>
> 1/2 teaspoon grated lemon peel
>
> 24 cherrystone or littleneck clams, scrubbed
>
> Hot-pepper sauce (optional)

Preheat the grill.

In a small cup, combine the parsley, garlic, and lemon peel.

Place the clams on the grill rack over medium-hot coals and cook for 5 minutes, or until the shells open. Remove with tongs. Discard any unopened clams. Sprinkle the parsley mixture over the clams. Serve with hot-pepper sauce, if using.

Makes 4 servings

NUTRITION AT A GLANCE

Per serving: 45 calories, 1/2 g fat, 0 g saturated fat, 7 g protein, 2 g carbohydrate, 0 g dietary fiber, 20 mg cholesterol, 30 mg sodium

Salmon Ball

Pick out the veggies of your choosing, and hit a home run with our salmon ball.

2	cups canned salmon, drained, flaked, and skin and bones removed
8	ounces reduced-fat cream cheese, softened
1	tablespoon finely chopped onion
1	tablespoon lemon juice
1	teaspoon prepared horseradish
1/4	teaspoon salt
1/4	teaspoon liquid smoke
1/2	cup chopped almonds
3	tablespoons chopped parsley

In a large bowl, combine the salmon, cream cheese, onion, lemon juice, horseradish, salt, and liquid smoke; mix thoroughly. Refrigerate for 4 hours, or until firm enough to form into a ball.

In a small bowl, combine the almonds and parsley. Shape the salmon mixture into a ball. Roll in the almond mixture. Refrigerate for 1 hour, or until chilled.

Makes one 5-inch ball (sixteen 2-tablespoon servings)

NUTRITION AT A GLANCE

Per serving: 80 calories, 5 g fat, 1 1/2 g saturated fat, 6 g protein, 2 g carbohydrate, 0 g dietary fiber, 15 mg cholesterol, 190 mg sodium

From the Menu of . . .

CASA TUA RESTAURANT

1700 St. James Avenue, Miami Beach

CHEF SERGIO SIGALA

Casa Tua is a beautiful restaurant in a converted European-style villa. This fabulous Tuna Tartare is Phase 3 with bread but Phase 1 if served with cucumbers instead.

Casa Tua Restaurant Tuna Tartare

PHASF 1

- 2 pounds tuna, sushi quality, chopped
- 1 ounce capers in salt, rinsed
- 6 ounces olives niçoise, pitted and cubed
- 4 ounces sun-dried tomatoes, cubed
- 2 tablespoons chopped cilantro
- 1 tablespoon chopped fresh red chile pepper (wear plastic gloves when handling)
- 1/2 cup Ligurian extra virgin olive oil
- 2 tablespoons balsamic vinegar

1 tablespoon Fleur de sel (French sea salt) or
  kosher salt

Mix the tuna, capers, olives, tomatoes, cilantro, and pepper, and season with the oil, vinegar, and Fleur de sel.

Note: Serve with grilled or toasted French bread or cucumber slices.

Makes 8 servings

NUTRITION AT A GLANCE

Per serving: 370 calories, 23 g fat, 2 1/2 g saturated fat, 30 g protein, 11 g carbohydrate, 2 g dietary fiber, 0 mg cholesterol, 1,460 mg sodium

Entertaining, South Beach-Style

Planning a party menu around a weight loss regimen may not seem like the most festive thing you'll ever do. But as Miami's top chefs have demonstrated, South Beach–legal dishes can be done in high culinary style, as you can see by the chef recipes sprinkled throughout the book. The diet offers lots of options for food to serve while entertaining at home, too.

We discussed this with Susan Kleinberg, a well-known Miami-area party planner, who came up with several ways to accommodate the diet at social events. If you're having a cocktail hour, you'll probably want finger food. Serve fresh vegetables, either raw or grilled with olive oil, with a low-fat or fat-free dip. Bowls of cashews or other nuts are a party staple. Try shrimp poached, steamed, or grilled. Smoked salmon with reduced-fat cream cheese on a whole grain cracker or pumpernickel square is another favorite. You can even go all the way to caviar and still be well within the guidelines.

If you're serving a buffet dinner, you'll want two or three entrées to choose from. A seared tuna fillet or a grilled salmon are great selections. Both can be prepared ahead of time and served at room temperature. Another good choice is roasted turkey breast or chicken breast in a Dijon mustard sauce. You can serve marinated flank steak for red-meat fans. All of these main courses are fine on the South Beach Diet.

For side dishes, you can set up a salad bar with marinated vegetables, various greens, and fresh toss-ins, including reduced-fat cheeses, fruits, and nuts. In place of the usual salad carbs such as croutons or pasta, offer salad made with tabbouleh, cracked bulgur wheat, or barley. You can even have pita bread with hummus on the side.

For dessert, you can create a beautiful berry bar, offering strawberries, blueberries, or whatever else is in season, accompanied by a bowl of shaved dark chocolate. Or you might serve melted dark chocolate and large strawberries on skewers for dipping. A dollop of whipped cream doesn't seem completely out of order, considering how virtuous you've been with the rest of the party menu.

Sun-Dried Tomato Tartlets with Cheeses

Widely used in Greek cuisine, phyllo is a thin, delicate dough that becomes light, airy, and flaky when baked. You can buy it fresh in Greek markets, but it's also available frozen in the supermarket. The frozen variety keeps for up to a year in the freezer.

8 sheets (17" × 11") frozen phyllo dough, thawed

3/4 cup (6 ounces) reduced-fat ricotta cheese

3 tablespoons reduced-fat crumbled goat cheese or reduced-fat feta cheese

1 egg white

1 scallion, chopped

2 tablespoons chopped fresh basil

2 cloves garlic, minced

1 1/2 ounces oil-packed sun-dried tomatoes, drained and chopped

Sprigs basil, for garnish

Preheat the oven to 375°F. Coat 24 miniature muffin cups with cooking spray.

Place 1 phyllo sheet on a work surface. Coat with cooking spray. Top with 3 more sheets, coating each sheet with cooking spray. Cut the sheets in thirds lengthwise and then in quarters crosswise to get 12 squares. Press each square into a muffin cup to form a shell with jagged edges. Repeat with the remaining sheets to line the remaining muffin cups.

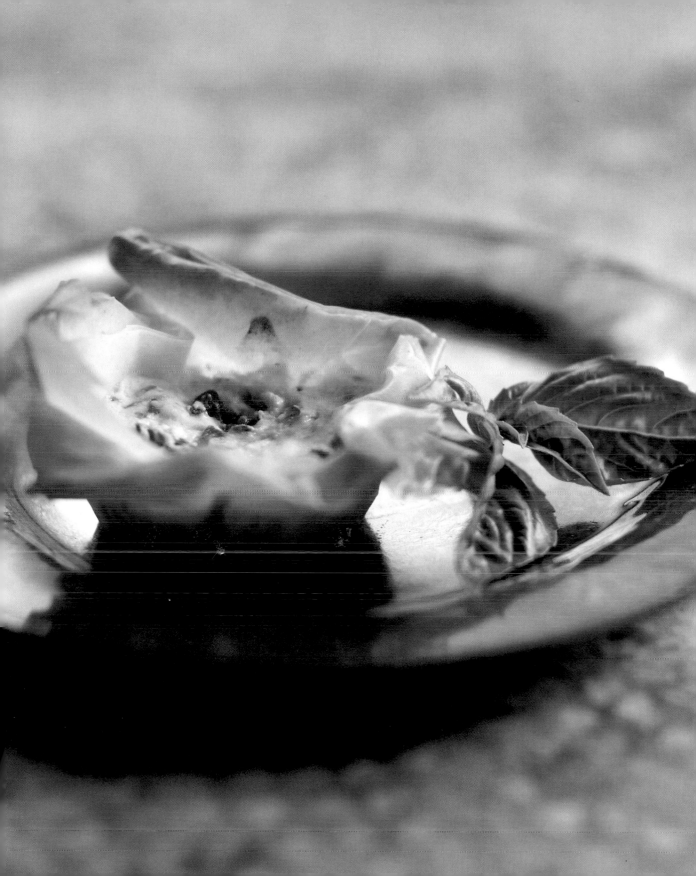

Bake for 5 minutes, or until golden.

Meanwhile in a food processor, combine the ricotta cheese, goat cheese or feta cheese, and egg white. Process until smooth. Add the scallion, basil, garlic, and tomatoes. Pulse briefly to mix. Spoon into the tart shells. Bake for 5 minutes, or until lightly puffed and heated through. Garnish with the basil sprigs.

Makes 24 tartlets

NUTRITION AT A GLANCE

Per 3 tartlets: 100 calories, 3 1/2 g fat, 1 1/2 g saturated fat, 5 g protein, 13 g carbohydrate, 0 g dietary fiber, 5 mg cholesterol, 200 mg sodium

Baked Tomatoes with Crab

Fresh lump crabmeat on juicy ripe tomatoes makes a rich and luscious combination. These savory treats are easy to make and bake in just 15 minutes, though their elegant appearance suggests otherwise!

1/2	cup finely ground nuts, such as pecans or walnuts
2	large tomatoes, halved
1	cup fresh lump crabmeat, well-drained
1	cup (4 ounces) shredded reduced-fat Monterey Jack cheese
1/2	cup black olives, finely chopped
1/2	cup mushrooms, finely chopped
1/2	cup parsley, finely chopped
1	clove garlic, minced
1/2	teaspoon dried oregano
1/2	teaspoon dried basil

Preheat the oven to 350°F. Coat a baking sheet with cooking spray.

Place the ground nuts on a plate. Coat both sides of the tomato halves with cooking spray. Dip the cut sides into the nuts to coat well. Place the tomatoes, cut side up, on the prepared baking sheet.

In a large bowl, combine the crabmeat, cheese, olives, mushrooms, parsley, garlic, oregano, and basil. Evenly divide the crab mixture among the tomatoes. Bake for 15 minutes, or until hot and bubbly.

Makes 4 servings

NUTRITION AT A GLANCE

Per serving: 240 calories, 17 g fat, 5 g saturated fat, 15 g protein, 10 g carbohydrate, 3 g dietary fiber, 35 mg cholesterol, 480 mg sodium

Spiced Pickled Eggs

Planning a picnic? A long car ride? A summer day by the pool? Or maybe you just want something to go in your salad. For all those occasions and more, these eggs may just be what you're looking for.

12	large eggs
2	cups white vinegar
1	medium onion, sliced and separated into rings
2	tablespoons sugar substitute
1 1/2	teaspoons pickling spice
1	teaspoon salt

Carefully place the eggs in a large pot. Fill the pot with water until the eggs are completely covered with about 1" of extra water. Bring the water to a boil over high heat. Turn off the heat. Cover and let stand on the burner for 18 minutes. Remove the pan from the stovetop, and run cold water into the pot until all the water is cool. Remove the eggs from the pan and refrigerate until cool.

Peel the eggs, place loosely in a large pickling jar, and set aside.

In a large saucepan, combine the vinegar, onion, sugar substitute, pickling spice, and salt. Bring to a boil over high heat. Reduce the heat to low heat and simmer for 5 minutes. Pour the hot mixture over the eggs, then seal with an airtight lid. Refrigerate the eggs until serving.

Makes 12 eggs

NUTRITION AT A GLANCE

Per egg: 80 calories, 5 g fat, 1 1/2 g saturated fat, 6 g protein, 2 g carbohydrate, 0 g dietary fiber, 215 mg cholesterol, 130 mg sodium

PHASE 1

Cottage Cheese-Stuffed Celery

This is spicy, sharp, snappy, and smooth all in one bite.

- 1/2 cup reduced-fat cottage cheese
- 1 scallion, chopped
- 1/8 teaspoon prepared horseradish
- 1/8 teaspoon Worcestershire sauce
- Pinch of garlic powder
- 4 ribs celery, cut into 3" pieces
- Paprika, for garnish

In a small bowl, combine the cottage cheese, scallion, horseradish, Worcestershire sauce, and garlic; mix thoroughly. Spoon into the celery pieces. Sprinkle with the paprika.

Makes 4 servings

NUTRITION AT A GLANCE

Per serving: 35 calories, 1 1/2 g fat, 1 g saturated fat, 4 g protein, 3 g carbohydrate, 0 g dietary fiber, 5 mg cholesterol, 150 mg sodium

Reuben Wrap

You will have to have a "rye" sense of humor for this Reuben; you won't find any bread in our wrap!

 1 leaf cabbage

 1 slice reduced-fat Swiss cheese

 1 slice pastrami

 1 tablespoon grainy mustard or sugar-free Thousand Island dressing

 2 tablespoons prepackaged coleslaw mix or sauerkraut

Fan the cabbage leaf on a plate. Place the cheese on the cabbage leaf and top with the pastrami. Spread the mustard or dressing onto the pastrami. Add the coleslaw or sauerkraut. Roll up and secure with a wooden pick.

Makes 1 wrap

NUTRITION AT A GLANCE

Per wrap: 180 calories, 11 g fat, 3 1/2 g saturated fat, 11 g protein, 7 g carbohydrate, 2 g dietary fiber, 35 mg cholesterol, 880 mg sodium

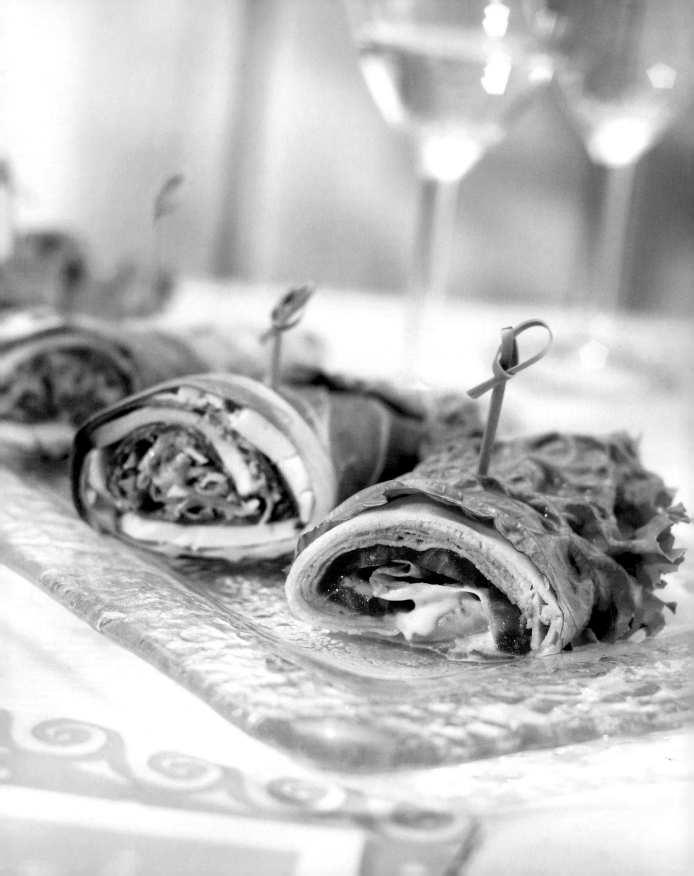

California Wrap

This is a great take-away snack. Prepare it the night before and wrap it tightly in plastic wrap to keep fresh for the next day.

1 leaf red or green lettuce

1 slice turkey breast

1 slice ham

1 thin slice tomato

1 thin slice avocado

1 teaspoon lime juice

1 leaf watercress or arugula

1 tablespoon sugar-free Ranch dressing

Fan the lettuce leaf on a plate. Top with the turkey, ham, and tomato.

In a small bowl, combine the avocado and lime juice, then spoon onto the tomato. Top with the watercress or arugula and dressing. Roll up and secure with a wooden pick.

Makes 1 wrap

NUTRITION AT A GLANCE

Per wrap: 140 calories, 10 g fat, 1 1/2 g saturated fat, 9 g protein, 4 g carbohydrate, 1 g dietary fiber, 25 mg cholesterol, 620 mg sodium

Muenster and Turkey Roll-Ups with Nut Butter

For a Phase 2 snack, you can add the optional apple slices to these roll-ups.

- 4 thin slices Swiss or Muenster cheese, at room temperature
- 2 ounces thinly sliced turkey breast
- 1/2 large apple, peeled and thinly sliced (optional for Phase 2)
- 1 tablespoon macadamia nut butter or 2 teaspoons unsweetened natural peanut butter

Place the cheese on a cutting board. Place the turkey on top. Add the apples, if using. Drizzle or spread with the nut butter or peanut butter and roll up. Secure with toothpicks.

Makes 4 roll-ups

NUTRITION AT A GLANCE

Per roll-up: 90 calories, 6 g fat, 3 g saturated fat, 7 g protein, 2 g carbohydrate, 0 g dietary fiber, 20 mg cholesterol, 220 mg sodium

Peanut Dip

If you want to have a little something to go with your raw veggies, this accompaniment is just what you've been looking for.

> 2 cups chopped unsalted roasted peanuts
> 1/2 cup fat-free plain yogurt
> 1/4 teaspoon finely grated lemon peel
> Salt

In a blender or food processor, combine the peanuts, yogurt, lemon peel, and salt to taste, and process until smooth.

Makes 2 1/2 cups

NUTRITION AT A GLANCE

Per tablespoon: 80 calories, 7 g fat, 1 g saturated fat, 4 g protein, 3 g carbohydrate, 0 g dietary fiber, 0 mg cholesterol, 0 mg sodium

Perky Ham Roll-Ups

Feel free to substitute any sugar-free preserve in this recipe, and if you want to add a little lettuce, go right ahead.

> 8 slices baked ham
>
> 1/2 cup sugar-free cherry preserves

Preheat the oven to 375°F.

Roll the ham slices and place in a shallow baking pan. Bake for 5 minutes, or until heated through.

Place the preserves in a microwaveable dish, cover, and microwave on medium for 30 seconds. Stir the preserves. If they are not hot enough, cover them and microwave for an additional 15 seconds.

Place 2 ham rolls on each of 4 serving plates. Drizzle each serving with the hot preserves.

Makes 8 roll-ups

NUTRITION AT A GLANCE

Per 2 roll-ups: 90 calories, 6 g fat, 3 g saturated fat, 7 g protein, 2 g carbohydrate, 0 g dietary fiber, 20 mg cholesterol, 220 mg sodium

Roasted Chickpeas

Can you enjoy a high-protein snack without meat or cheese? With the South Beach Diet you can.

1 can (14–19 ounces) chickpeas, rinsed and drained

Preheat the oven to 350°F.

Spread the chickpeas on an ungreased baking sheet in a single layer. Bake for 50 minutes, or until browned and crisp enough to rattle.

Makes 4 servings

NUTRITION AT A GLANCE

Per serving: 70 calories, 1 g fat, 0 g saturated fat, 4 g protein, 11 g carbohydrate, 3 g dietary fiber, 0 mg cholesterol, 10 mg sodium

From the Menu of . . .
THE FORGE
432 Arthur Godfrey Road, Miami Beach

CHEF ANDREW ROTHSCHILD

The Forge has been a landmark Miami restaurant for decades. But this mushroom "soup" is anything but outdated!

Wild Mushroom Cappuccino
PHASE 1

1   onion, diced

2   cloves garlic, crushed

2   tablespoons canola oil

2   cups of sliced assorted wild mushrooms (shiitake, cremini, cèpe)

1   quart roasted or plain chicken broth

1   ounce fresh thyme leaves or bunch of thyme stems

1   bay leaf

    Salt

    Pepper

1   cup cold fat-free milk

1   teaspoon porcini powder

Sauté onion and garlic in oil until translucent. Add mushrooms and sauté until they begin to caramelize. Add broth, thyme, and bay leaf. Reduce to half. Use a chinois (a fine, mesh sieve) to strain the mixture. Season with salt and pepper.

Pour into coffee cups. Froth cold milk on cappuccino machine. Spoon froth on top and sprinkle with the porcini powder.

Makes 4 servings

NUTRITION AT A GLANCE

Per serving: 170 calories, 11 g fat, 1 1/2 g saturated fat, 5 g protein, 13 g carbohydrate, 2 g dietary fiber, 5 mg cholesterol, 1,110 mg sodium

Black Bean Dip

Need something easy to please the kids? Or a quick party dip? This one's a hit every time. It's excellent with fresh vegetables or whole wheat pita crisps on Phase 2. It's best hot, but it's good cold as well.

  1 can (14–19 ounces) fat-free refried black or pinto beans
  1 cup fat-free sour cream
  1 can (14 1/2 ounces) diced tomatoes
  1 jalapeño chile pepper, chopped (wear plastic gloves when handling)
1/2 teaspoon salt
  1 teaspoon ground black pepper
  1 cup (4 ounces) shredded reduced-fat Cheddar cheese (optional)

Preheat the oven to 325°F.

In a large bowl, combine the beans, sour cream, tomatoes (with juice), chile pepper, salt, and black pepper. Spoon into a 1-quart shallow baking dish or pie plate. Top with the cheese, if using.

Bake for 10 minutes, or until heated through.

Makes 3 cups

NUTRITION AT A GLANCE

Per 2 tablespoons: 45 calories, 2 1/2 g fat, 1 1/2 g saturated fat, 3 g protein, 4 g carbohydrate, 1 g dietary fiber, 10 mg cholesterol, 140 mg sodium

Tomato Salsa with Avocado and Onion

Easy to prepare, a salsa like this is a refreshing appetizer with tasty dippers, or it's a sassy addition to plain chicken, fish, or vegetables. Serve with toasted whole wheat pita triangles for a Phase 2 snack.

2 tomatoes, finely chopped

1/2 red onion, chopped

1/4 avocado, cubed

1 green chile pepper, seeded and chopped (wear plastic gloves when handling)

2 tablespoons chopped parsley

1 tablespoon red wine vinegar

2 teaspoons grated lime peel

1 teaspoon lime juice

1/4 teaspoon ground cumin

Assorted cut fresh vegetables, such as celery sticks, cauliflower florets, or cucumber slices

Whole wheat pita triangles (see note)

In a large serving bowl, combine the tomatoes, onion, avocado, pepper, parsley, vinegar, lime peel, lime juice, and cumin. Let stand for 15 minutes before serving. Serve with the cut vegetables for dipping and pita triangles.

Note: To make the pita triangles, cut pita in triangles and bake in 350°F oven until lightly browned.

Makes 6 servings

NUTRITION AT A GLANCE

Per serving: 100 calories, 2 g fat, 0 g saturated fat, 3 g protein, 18 g carbohydrate, 4 g dietary fiber, 0 mg cholesterol, 135 mg sodium

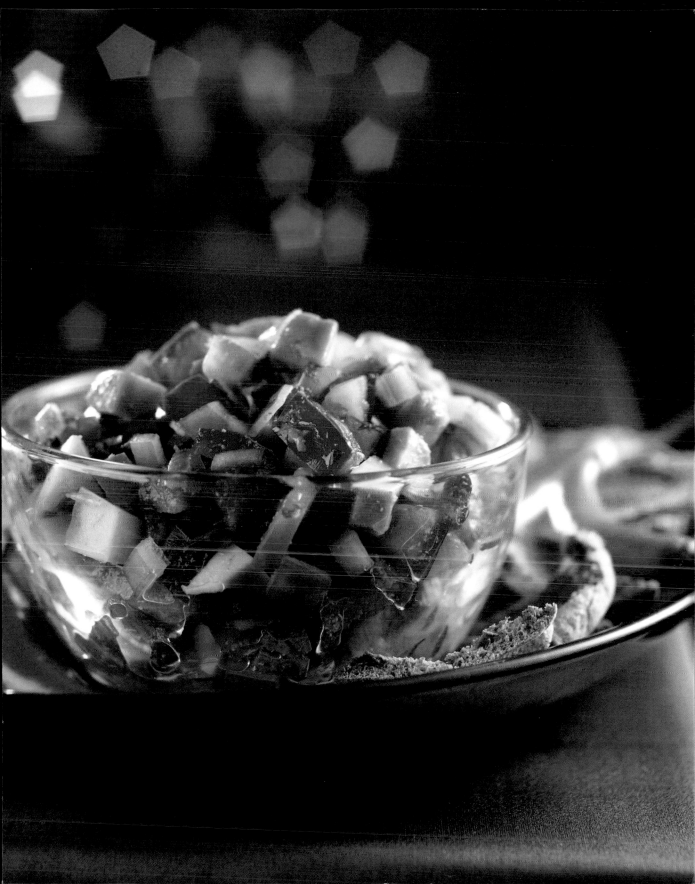

Yogurt Cheese Cucumber Dip

You can easily make a satiny cream cheese from yogurt. It is delicious plain or mixed with chopped chives or garlic and stuffed into mushroom caps or cherry tomatoes. Here it's combined with a refreshing cucumber mixture to make a satisfying dip you can scoop up with fresh vegetables. This recipe is a favorite of my sister, Alice.

2	cups fat-free plain yogurt
1	cucumber, grated
1/2	cup fresh lemon juice
2	cloves garlic, minced
1	tablespoon chopped fresh dill

Line a strainer or sieve with a double layer of cheesecloth and place it over a bowl. Spoon in the yogurt and tie the corners of the cheesecloth together. Let it drain in the refrigerator overnight. Do not allow the strainer to touch the liquid. Squeeze the yogurt gently and remove it from the cheesecloth. Discard the liquid or reserve for another use. Use immediately or cover and refrigerate for up to 5 days.

Squeeze the cucumber in a towel to remove the moisture.

In a large bowl, combine the cucumber, yogurt cheese, lemon juice, and garlic. Sprinkle with the dill.

Makes 1 cup

NUTRITION AT A GLANCE

Per 2 tablespoons: 40 calories, 0 g fat, 0 g saturated fat, 3 g protein, 7 g carbohydrate, 0 g dietary fiber, 0 mg cholesterol, 35 mg sodium

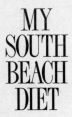

MY SOUTH BEACH DIET

THIS NEW WAY OF EATING HAS LITERALLY SAVED MY LIFE.

The South Beach Diet has saved my life. At 38 years old and 400 pounds, I was desperate to make a change and seriously considering gastric bypass surgery—until I learned about the South Beach Diet.

What really triggered me to lose weight was my partner of 17 years, Dennis. His support is unmatched, and I knew that if I didn't do something about my weight, we wouldn't have many more years to spend with each other.

I started Phase 1 on June 23. At that time, my cholesterol was 280, my triglycerides were 248, and my blood pressure was 165/95, even with medication. Then in September, I went back to my doctor for a checkup. My weight had dropped to 347 pounds. My cholesterol was 177, my triglycerides were 105, and my blood pressure was down to 126/70. All my doctor could say was "Phenomenal . . . phenomenal . . . phenomenal. . . . "

Luckily, I found this new way of life pretty easy from the start. I stayed on Phase 1 for 3 weeks and lost 32 pounds, just by following the food suggestions presented in the book. The dramatic weight loss in such a short period of time motivated me to keep going.

I felt good about South Beach because I was learning the right way to fuel my body. I learned how important it is to eat three meals a day with three snacks in between and that the way to lose weight was not skipping meals. It was strange eating a snack when I wasn't very hungry, but I soon realized the importance of it. It kept me from getting famished and overeating later in the day.

In Phase 2, I added whole grain bread, pita bread, whole grain pasta, berries, and, yes, chocolate back into my diet. I've continued to lose weight at the rate of 1 to 2 pounds a week. Recently, I started walking and now walk 1 mile, three times each day. I lost 4 pounds last week, and my total weight loss after being on the South Beach Diet for only 3 months is now 57 pounds!

This new way of eating has literally saved my life. I really believe I'm learning a sensible way to eat that I can live with forever. My partner is also extremely proud of what I have accomplished so far. I now know we'll have many more years to share together.

Not only do I know I will reach my goal weight, but I also know I'll keep it off this time. —*EDWARD O*.

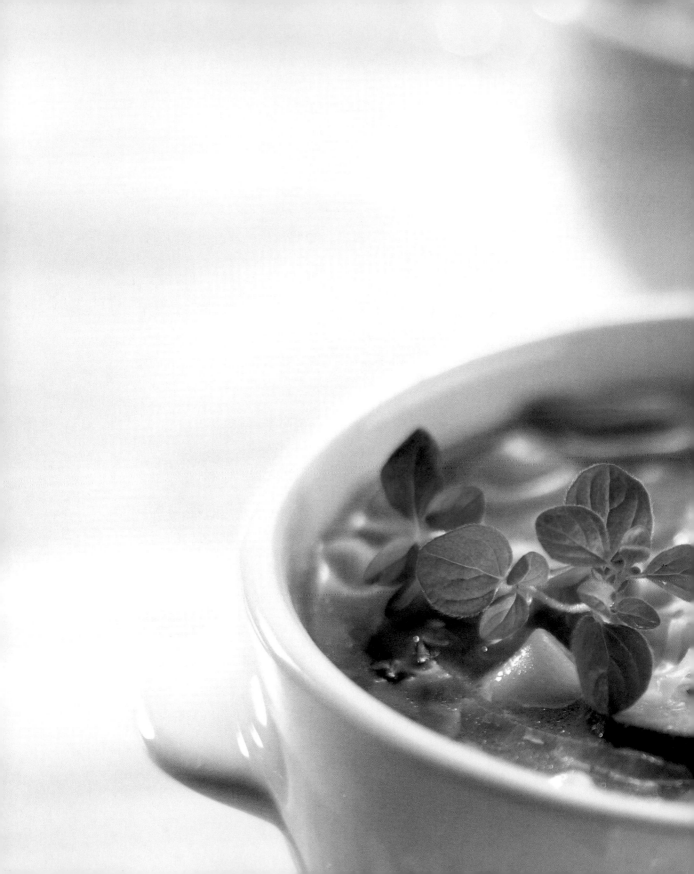

SOUPS

Here's why soup is a good idea for dieters: The human brain doesn't even begin getting the message that you're filling your belly until 20 minutes or so after you've begun to eat. So any low-carb first course is good because it starts sending the message early. When served as an appetizer, soup extends the overall meal time and automatically keeps you from stuffing yourself later in the meal.

In Phase 1 of the diet, I recommend either chicken or beef broth-based soup, gazpacho, or soups with lots of vegetables. After those 2 weeks, nearly all soups are South Beach–legal, either as an appetizer or as a main course. There's no end to the combinations of meat, fish, vegetables, and whole grains you can use. You may even include modest amounts of whole wheat pasta or long-cooking rice. I've included several recipes for thick, creamy soups made without cream. You'll never miss it!

Asian-Style Gazpacho

Serve this clever combination of ingredients as a light first course with any variety of other dishes. It's also perfect for a light summer lunch out on the porch.

- 6 tomatoes, seeded and finely chopped
- 2 cups chicken broth
- 1 teaspoon dry sherry
- 2 tablespoons chopped fresh cilantro
- 1 tablespoon light soy sauce
- 4 scallions, white part only
- 4 thin slices fresh ginger
- 1/4 teaspoon Chinese chili sauce
- 2 limes

Place the tomatoes in a 2- or 3-quart saucepan over low heat. Add the broth, sherry, cilantro, soy sauce, scallions, and ginger. Bring the mixture to a simmer and cook for 20 minutes. Remove from the heat and allow to cool for a few minutes. Puree in a food processor or blender. Chill.

Right before serving, stir in the chili sauce. Grate the peel from 1 lime and add it to the soup. Squeeze the juice from both limes into the soup. Serve in chilled bowls.

Makes 6 servings

NUTRITION AT A GLANCE

Per serving: 48 calories, 1 g fat, 0 g saturated fat, 2 g protein, 9 g carbohydrate, 2 g dietary fiber, 0 mg cholesterol, 454 mg sodium

Chilled Tomato Bisque

If you want something easy, try this tomato bisque. It's rich and creamy and quite tasty.

4	medium tomatoes, peeled, seeded, and finely chopped
1 1/2	cups V8 juice or vegetable cocktail juice
1	cup buttermilk
1	teaspoon dried basil
1/4	teaspoon ground black pepper

Place the tomatoes, V8 juice or vegetable cocktail juice, buttermilk, basil, and pepper in a blender or food processor and process until smooth. Refrigerate for at least 1 hour before serving.

Makes 4 servings

NUTRITION AT A GLANCE
Per serving: 71 calories, 1 g fat, 0 g saturated fat, 4 g protein, 13 g carbohydrate, 2 g dietary fiber, 2 mg cholesterol, 308 mg sodium

PICASSO

The Bellagio Hotel, 3600 Las Vegas Boulevard,
South Las Vegas

EXECUTIVE CHEF
JULIAN SERRANO

WHILE *PICASSO* IS NOT IN MIAMI, CHEF JULIAN SERRANO IS
A PART OF THE ANNUAL SOUTH BEACH WINE AND FOOD
FESTIVAL. IT'S ONE OF MY FAVORITE LOCAL EVENTS.

Classic Gazpacho with Avocado Crab Farci
PHASE 3

Gazpacho

1 1/2	pounds ripe tomatoes, cut in pieces (reserve 1/2 tomato for stuffing)
1/2	large green bell pepper, chopped
1/2	medium onion, chopped
1/2	cucumber, seeded and chopped
2	cloves garlic
2	cups tomato juice
1	tablespoon whole cumin
4	tablespoons sherry vinegar

4	slices day-old bread
2	cups water
2	tablespoons extra virgin olive oil
	Salt
	Pepper

Stuffed Avocado

2	Haas (California) avocados, halved
1/2	cucumber, seeded and finely chopped
1/2	onion, finely chopped
1/2	tomato, finely chopped (reserved from gazpacho)
1/2	green bell pepper, finely chopped
1	pound lump crabmeat
	Cherry tomatoes, for garnish

To make the gazpacho: Put the tomatoes, bell pepper, onion, cucumber, garlic, tomato juice, cumin, vinegar, bread, water, and oil in a large bowl for 6 hours. After 6 hours, put the ingredients in a blender and blend well. Season with salt and pepper to taste. Refrigerate until cold.

To make the stuffed avocados: Remove the flesh of each avocado half, leaving a 1/2" shell around each.

In a small bowl, mix the avocado flesh, cucumber, onion, tomato, and pepper. Divide the mixture into the avocado halves. Top each avocado half with crabmeat.

Serve in chilled bowls. Put 1/2 the stuffed avocado in center of each bowl with gazpacho ladled around. Garnish each serving with cherry tomatoes.

Makes 4 servings

NUTRITION AT A GLANCE

Per serving: 431 calories, 23 g fat, 3 1/2 g saturated fat, 25 g protein, 37 g carbohydrate, 12 g dietary fiber, 85 mg cholesterol, 520 mg sodium

Indian Tomato Soup

This fragrant and spicy tomato soup makes for an interesting beginning to any meal. If you don't want to blanch the tomatoes, you can use canned crushed tomatoes instead.

1/2 pound red vine-ripened tomatoes or 1 (16 ounce) can crushed tomatoes, undrained

2 tablespoons extra virgin olive oil

1 medium onion, finely chopped

1 green chile pepper, seeded and finely chopped (wear plastic gloves when handling)

3 cloves garlic, crushed

1 tablespoon tomato paste

4 cups vegetable broth

1/2 teaspoon curry powder

Chopped fresh cilantro, for garnish

If using fresh tomatoes, bring a large pot of water deep enough to submerge the tomatoes to a boil over high heat. Cut a small ✗ in the bottom of each tomato and plunge them into the boiling water for 30 seconds each. Remove the tomatoes. When cool enough to handle, peel away the loosened skin. If the skin fails to peel away easily, return the tomatoes to the boiling water for an additional 10 seconds. Remove the cores from the tomatoes and coarsely chop the flesh.

Heat the oil in a large saucepan over medium heat. Add the onion, chile pepper, and garlic and cook for 4 minutes, or until soft. Stir in the fresh or canned tomatoes and cook, stirring often, for 5 minutes.

In a small bowl, blend the tomato paste with the vegetable broth and add to the saucepan. Add the curry powder and simmer for 7 minutes.

To serve, divide the soup among 4 serving bowls. Sprinkle the cilantro on top for garnish.

Makes 4 servings

NUTRITION AT A GLANCE

Per serving: 122 calories, 8 g fat, 1 g saturated fat, 4 g protein, 12 g carbohydrate, 2 g dietary fiber, 0 mg cholesterol, 1,015 mg sodium

Teriyaki Mushroom Soup with Watercress

Watercress is actually a member of the mustard family, and it has a slightly bitter flavor that is tempered here with teriyaki sauce, lemon juice, and fresh cilantro. If you eliminate the cellophane noodles and prepare the South Beach Teriyaki Sauce (see recipe on page 241), you can also enjoy this recipe in Phase 1.

        4 cups chicken broth
        1 tablespoon teriyaki sauce
    2 1/2 cups thinly sliced mushrooms
        2 cups watercress, finely chopped
        1 package (3 1/2 ounces) cellophane noodles
        1 tablespoon lemon juice
        1 tablespoon chopped fresh cilantro
           Pinch of ground red pepper

Bring the broth and teriyaki sauce to a boil in a 3-quart saucepan over medium-high heat. Reduce the heat to low and stir in the mushrooms, watercress, noodles, lemon juice, cilantro, and red pepper. Simmer for 7 minutes, or until the noodles and mushrooms are tender.

Makes 6 servings

NUTRITION AT A GLANCE

Per serving: 90 calories, 1 g fat, 0 g saturated fat, 3 g protein, 17 g carbohydrate, 1 g dietary fiber, 0 mg cholesterol, 787 mg sodium

Peanut Butter Stew

About 75 percent of all American homes have a jar of peanut butter on the shelf. If you're peanutty for peanut butter's taste, you'll be nutty for this stew. It's great for lunch or dinner.

      2 tablespoons peanut oil

      1 large onion, finely chopped

      2 pounds round steak, cut into 1 1/2" pieces

    1/2 cup creamy unsweetened natural peanut butter

  1 1/2 cups cold water

    1/3 cup double-strength tomato concentrate
         (Italian tube)

      2 cups hot water

      1 teaspoon chipotle pepper powder

      2 bay leaves
         Salt
         Freshly ground black pepper

Heat the oil in a heavy saucepan over medium heat. Add the onion and cook for 3 minutes, or until the onion is translucent. Add the steak and cook, stirring occasionally, for 5 minutes, or until the meat is lightly browned on all sides.

In a small bowl, combine the peanut butter with the cold water, then pour it over the meat. Dilute the tomato concentrate with the hot water and pour over the stew. Stir thoroughly. Add the chipotle pepper powder, bay leaves, and salt and black pepper to taste. Reduce the heat to low, cover, and cook, stirring occasionally, for 1 hour, or until the meat is tender. Remove and discard the bay leaves. Serve hot.

Makes 6 servings

NUTRITION AT A GLANCE

Per serving: 444 calories, 27 g fat, 7 g saturated fat, 40 g protein, 10 g carbohydrate, 3 g dietary fiber, 9 mg cholesterol, 308 mg sodium

PHASE 1 ## Walnut Soup

*A soup is a soup, but this one has all the ingredients
of a meal.*

- 1 large bulb fennel, cut into quarters
- 2 tablespoons extra virgin olive oil
  Kosher salt
  Freshly ground black pepper
- 1 leek, white part only, sliced
- 1 cup cauliflower florets
- 2 cups chicken broth
- 1/2 cup fat-free half and half
- 2 tablespoons dry sherry
- 1/2 cup coarsely chopped toasted walnuts
- 1/4 cup crumbled Stilton or Roquefort cheese
  Finely chopped lemon peel
- 1 tablespoon chopped fresh chives

Preheat the oven to 400°F.

In a large baking pan, toss the fennel with 1
tablespoon of the oil and sprinkle with the salt and
pepper to taste. Bake for 15 minutes, or until tender
and golden brown. When cool enough to handle, slice
into 1/2" strips.

Meanwhile, heat the remaining 1 tablespoon oil in a
heavy medium-size pot over medium-low heat. Add
the leek, stirring until coated with oil. Cover and cook
for 5 minutes, or until the leeks are translucent. Add

the cauliflower and broth and bring to a boil. Reduce the heat to low and simmer for 20 minutes, or until the cauliflower is tender. Remove the mixture to a blender or food processor. Add the fennel to the blender or food processor. Process to puree until smooth and return to the pot. Add the half and half and sherry. Return to a simmer while stirring in the walnuts.

In a small bowl, combine the cheese and lemon peel. Serve the soup in warmed bowls, adding the cheese and chives immediately before serving.

Makes 4 servings

NUTRITION AT A GLANCE
Per serving: 244 calories, 21 g fat, 4 g saturated fat, 7 g protein, 10 g carbohydrate, 4 g dietary fiber, 8 mg cholesterol, 694 mg sodium

From the Menu of . . .
TALULA RESTAURANT & BAR
210 23rd Street, Miami Beach

CHEFS ANDREA CURTO-RANDAZZO AND FRANK RANDAZZO

TALULA IS A WARM AND INVITING SPACE, AND ITS OWNERS SAY IT WAS DESIGNED TO FEEL LIKE THEIR HOME. NOW YOU CAN ENJOY THEIR FOOD IN *YOUR* HOME.

Roasted Yellow Pepper Soup with Fava Beans and Teardrop Tomatoes
PHASE 1

Soup

5	yellow bell peppers
2	tablespoons extra virgin olive oil
1	teaspoon salt
1/2	large Vidalia onion, chopped
3	cloves garlic, sliced
2	teaspoons ancho chile powder
1 1/4	quarts vegetable or chicken broth
	Ground white pepper

Garnish

- 1 cup fresh fava beans in pods or 1 cup canned fava beans (rinsed and drained)
- 2 teaspoons salt
- 1 tablespoon extra virgin olive oil
- 1 cup red teardrop tomatoes, halved lengthwise
- 1 tablespoon chives, finely chopped

  Juice of 1/2 lemon

  Pinch salt

  Pinch pepper

To make the soup: Preheat the oven to 350°F.

Wash peppers and place in a large bowl. Toss in 1 tablespoon olive oil and 1 teaspoon salt. Place on a baking sheet and roast in the oven until blistered and brown, about 15 minutes. Remove from the oven and let cool.

In large heavy-gauge pot, sauté the onion and garlic in 1 tablespoon olive oil on medium heat until tender, about 5 to 7 minutes, stirring frequently.

Peel the peppers and remove all seeds. Add peppers and ancho

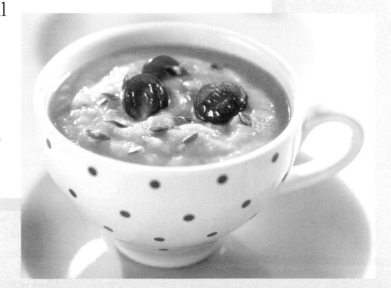

powder to onions and garlic. Bring heat up to high and sauté for 1 minute. Add the broth and bring to a boil. Turn heat to medium-low and simmer for 25 to 30 minutes, stirring occasionally.

Puree the soup with a hand mixer or in a blender until smooth. Strain through a china cap or cheesecloth-lined strainer and season with salt and white pepper to taste.

To make the garnish: Remove the fava beans from their pods.

While the soup is simmering, bring 4 cups water and 2 teaspoons salt to a boil. Add the fava beans and cook until tender, about 3 minutes. Remove, strain, and shock in ice water to prevent overcooking. Once cool, drain and remove outer casing from beans. Set aside.

Ladle the soup into bowls. In a small sauté pan, on medium heat, add 1 tablespoon olive oil. Add the fava beans and sauté for 1 minute. Add the tomatoes, chives, lemon juice and a pinch of salt and pepper. Spoon the mixture into the middle of each serving.

Makes 6 servings

NUTRITION AT A GLANCE

Per serving: 92 calories, 4 g fat, 1 g saturated fat, 3 g protein, 13 g carbohydrate, 4 g dietary fiber, 0 mg cholesterol, 891 mg sodium

Hearty Minestrone

This recipe calls for ditalini or small shell pasta, but any other small, shaped pasta will work equally well. If you leave the pasta out, it's a Phase 1 dish.

1 tablespoon extra virgin olive oil

2 leeks, white and green parts, white halved lengthwise, rinsed and thinly sliced, green parts chopped

2 ribs celery with leaves, thinly sliced

2 cloves garlic, minced

1/4 teaspoon dried oregano, crushed

1/4 teaspoon ground black pepper

1/8 teaspoon salt

3 cups chicken broth

4 cups Swiss chard, chopped

1 cup green beans, cut into 1" pieces

1/4 cup whole wheat ditalini or small shell pasta

1 clove garlic, coarsely chopped

1/4 cup chopped Italian parsley

1/2 cup sliced zucchini

4 teaspoons grated Parmesan cheese

4 sprigs oregano, for garnish

Heat the oil in a large saucepan over medium heat. Add the leeks, celery, minced garlic, dried oregano, pepper, and salt. Cook, stirring frequently, for 4 minutes, or until the vegetables begin to soften.

Add the broth, Swiss chard, green beans, and pasta. Bring to a boil over high heat. Reduce the heat to medium-low, cover, and simmer for 8 minutes, or until the vegetables are tender and the pasta is al dente.

Meanwhile, in a cup, combine the chopped garlic with the parsley. Stir into the soup along with the zucchini. Cover and cook for 5 minutes, or until heated through.

Ladle the soup into 4 bowls and top each with 1 teaspoon of the cheese. Garnish with the oregano sprigs.

Makes 4 servings

NUTRITION AT A GLANCE

Per serving: 138 calories, 6 g fat, 1 g saturated fat, 5 g protein, 17 g carbohydrate, 3 g dietary fiber, 1 mg cholesterol, 988 mg sodium

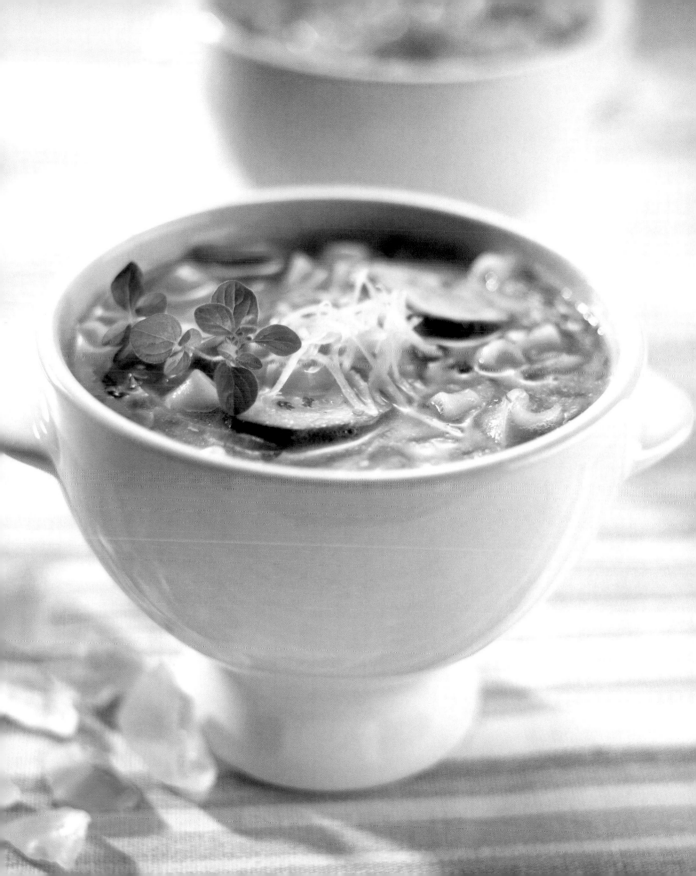

White Bean Soup with Greens

This southern Italian soup features white beans. Choose from great Northern beans, cannellini beans, or any other white bean you happen to have on hand.

1 1/2	pounds Swiss chard, escarole, or beet greens, trimmed
6	cups chicken broth
1	clove garlic, crushed
1	cup cooked white beans
1/2	teaspoon salt
1/8	teaspoon ground white pepper
	Grated Parmesan cheese, for garnish
	Red-pepper flakes, for garnish

Bring a large pot of water to a boil over medium-high heat. Add the greens and cook for 7 minutes, or until barely tender. Drain the greens, squeezing out as much water as possible. (This can be done several hours before cooking in the soup. It is not necessary to cut the greens, because they will break apart while they cook in the soup.)

Bring the broth to a simmer in a large pot over medium-high heat. Add the garlic and greens. If using canned white beans, place them in a strainer and rinse them under cold running water to remove excess sodium. Add the beans to the broth. Simmer gently, partially covered, for 10 minutes. Sprinkle with the salt and pepper to taste. (Do not add the salt before the soup has finished cooking, or it may become too salty.)

Ladle the soup into heated bowls. Pass the cheese and pepper flakes at the table.

Makes 6 servings

NUTRITION AT A GLANCE
Per serving: 79 calories, 2 g fat, 1 g saturated fat, 6 g protein, 12 g carbohydrate, 4 g dietary fiber, 0 mg cholesterol, 1,008 mg sodium

Black and White Bean Soup

This soup is truly a meal unto itself, with a heaping serving of both protein and fiber. Enjoy this soup with a crisp salad and a fresh pear for dessert.

3/4	cup dried black beans
3/4	cup dried great Northern beans
2	tablespoons extra virgin olive oil
1	medium onion, chopped
1	small poblano chile pepper, seeded and finely chopped (wear plastic gloves when handling)
1	small rib celery, chopped
4	cloves garlic, sliced
1 1/2	teaspoons chopped fresh thyme leaves
8	cups chicken broth
1	teaspoon chili powder
1	teaspoon ground cumin
1	teaspoon chopped fresh sage
	Roasted-Pepper Cream (see recipe on page 229)
	Fresh cilantro leaves, for garnish

Place black beans and great Northern beans in two separate large bowls, cover with cold water, and soak overnight in the refrigerator.

Heat the oil in a large pot over medium heat. Add the onion, chile pepper, celery, garlic, and thyme and cook for 8 minutes, or until the vegetables are tender. Remove half of the vegetables to another large pot.

Drain the beans. To the first pot, add the black beans, 4 cups of broth, the chili powder and the cumin. To the second pot, add the great Northern beans, the remaining 4 cups broth, and the sage. Heat both pots to boiling and cover. Reduce the heat to low. Simmer the black-bean pot for 1 1/2 hours and the white-bean pot for 1 hour. Keep both warm over low heat.

To serve, ladle 1 cup black bean soup into each of 4 serving bowls. Tilt the bowls and ladle 1 cup white-bean soup into the other side of each bowl. Drizzle with the Roasted-Pepper Cream and garnish with the cilantro leaves.

Makes 4 servings

NUTRITION AT A GLANCE

Per serving: 410 calories, 11 g fat, 2 g saturated fat, 23 g protein, 56 g carbohydrate, 14 g dietary fiber, 10 mg cholesterol, 410 mg sodium

From the Menu of . . .
JOE'S STONE CRAB
11 Washington Avenue, Miami Beach

CHEF ANDRE BIENVENU

If you're planning a trip to Miami, make sure you go during Stone Crab season (October 15–May 15) so you can eat at *Joe's*.

Manhattan Clam Chowder
PHASE 3

1/4	cup salt pork, chopped (optional)
2/3	cup potatoes, chopped
1/3	cup yellow onion, chopped
2/3	cup carrot, chopped
1/2	cup celery, chopped
4–5	cloves chopped garlic
6	ounces chopped clams (about 12 clams)
1/2	cup clam juice
1 1/4	cups canned diced tomatoes with juice
2	teaspoons tomato paste
2	teaspoons ketchup

1	teaspoon Magi seasoning
1/2	teaspoon dried thyme
2	tablespoons all-purpose flour
2	tablespoons cold water
1/2	ounce chopped green bell pepper (about 2 tablespoons)
	Salt
	Black pepper

Brown the salt pork in a kettle or pot until golden brown. Pour off excess fat. Add the potatoes and cook halfway. Add the onion, carrot, celery, garlic, clams, clam juice, diced tomatoes, tomato paste, ketchup, Magi seasoning, and thyme. Allow to cook for 20 minutes on simmer.

In a cup, mix the flour and water to make a paste. Add to the soup. Allow 5 minutes to cook out. Add the green peppers and cook for a few more minutes.

Add salt and black pepper to taste.

Makes 2 servings

NUTRITION AT A GLANCE

Per serving: 214 calories, 1 g fat, 0 g saturated fat, 18 g protein, 36 g carbohydrate, 6 g dietary fiber, 31 mg cholesterol, 567 mg sodium

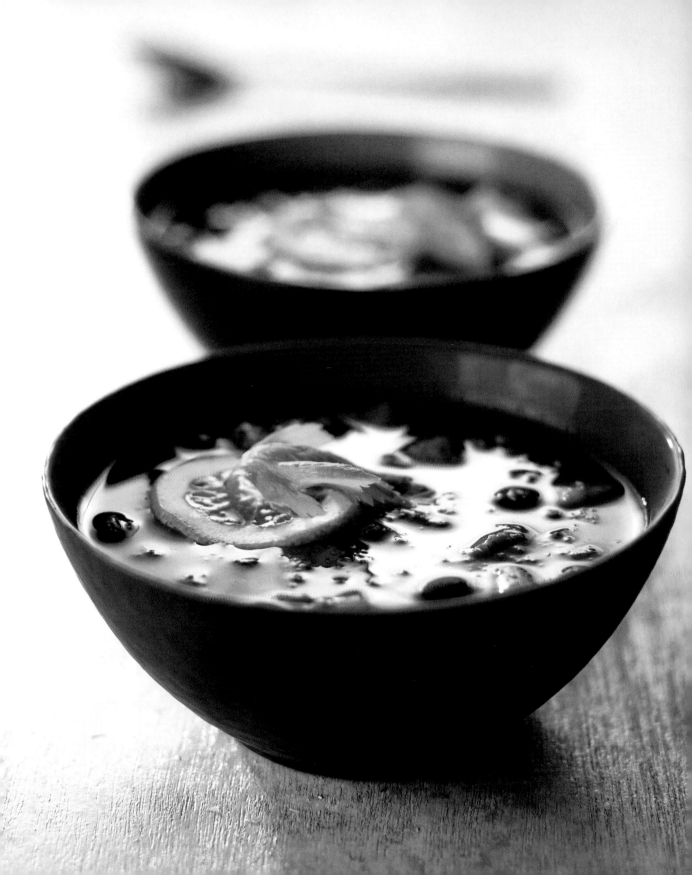

Black Bean Soup

This soup gets its inspiration from the Latin community. If you like, you can sprinkle a little bit of shredded reduced-fat Cheddar over the soup just before serving.

1 1/2   cups dried black beans

    6   cups water

    2   tablespoons extra virgin olive oil

    1   onion, chopped

    3   cloves garlic, minced

    1   rib celery, with leaves, chopped

        Ground black pepper

    1   teaspoon celery seeds

        Juice of 1 1/2 lemons

    1   lemon, sliced paper thin, for garnish

        Leaves celery, for garnish

Place the beans in a large bowl and cover with the water. Add more water if necessary to cover the beans. Soak overnight. Drain the beans and add 6 cups of fresh water to the bowl.

Heat the oil in a large heavy-bottomed pot over medium heat. Add the onion, garlic, and celery and cook, stirring occasionally, for 5 minutes, or until tender. Add the beans and water and bring to a boil. Reduce the heat to low, cover, and simmer for 2 hours, or until the beans are tender.

Remove half of the beans to a food processor or blender and process to puree, adding the liquid from the soup to cover. Add the black pepper to taste and the celery seeds. Return the pureed beans to the pot and heat, stirring, until the soup thickens. Stir in the lemon juice.

Ladle into 6 serving bowls, and garnish with the sliced lemon and celery leaves.

Makes 6 servings

NUTRITION AT A GLANCE

Per serving: 230 calories, 5 g fat, 1 g saturated fat, 11 g protein, 35 g carbohydrate, 8 g dietary fiber, 0 mg cholesterol, 15 mg sodium

Creole Gumbo

Creole cooking makes ample use of celery, onions, peppers, and tomatoes, and so did we.

2	tablespoons extra virgin olive oil
2	ribs celery, chopped
1/2	small onion, chopped
1/2	green bell pepper, chopped
2	cloves garlic, minced
1 1/2	tablespoons whole wheat flour
2	teaspoons salt
2/3	cup canned tomatoes
2/3	cup South Beach Tomato Sauce (see recipe on page 234)
1	tablespoon Worcestershire sauce
1	cup frozen okra, partially thawed and cut into 1/2" pieces
1	cup coarsely chopped shrimp
1	cup lump crabmeat, flaked
1/4	cup hot water
1	tablespoon finely chopped parsley

Heat the oil in a 5-quart saucepan over medium-high heat. Add the celery, onion, pepper, and garlic and cook, stirring occasionally, for 10 minutes, or until softened. Stir in the flour and salt and cook until the mixture bubbles. Add the tomatoes, South Beach Tomato Sauce, and Worcestershire sauce. Reduce the heat to low, cover, and simmer for 20 minutes. Add the okra, shrimp, crabmeat, water, and parsley and simmer for 20 minutes longer. Serve hot.

Makes 4 servings

NUTRITION AT A GLANCE

Per serving: 192 calories, 8 g fat, 3 g saturated fat, 16 g protein, 13 g carbohydrate, 3 g dietary fiber, 85 mg cholesterol, 901 mg sodium

Buttermilk Salmon Chowder

Yogurt and buttermilk add creaminess to this chunky chowder. Dill, bay leaf, and tarragon lend the perfect flavor accents.

2 turnips, peeled and cut into small cubes
1 onion, chopped
1 rib celery, chopped
1 teaspoon dill seed
1 bay leaf
2 cups vegetable broth or water
1 can (12 ounces) pink salmon, drained
1 cup buttermilk
1 cup (8 ounces) fat-free plain yogurt
1 tablespoon trans-free margarine
2 teaspoons hot-pepper sauce
1/4 teaspoon salt
1/2 teaspoon ground black pepper
1/4 teaspoon dried tarragon

In a large saucepan, combine the turnips, onion, celery, dill seed, bay leaf, and broth or water. Bring to a boil over high heat. Reduce the heat to medium and simmer for 12 minutes, or until the vegetables are tender.

Reduce the heat to low. Stir in the salmon, buttermilk, yogurt, margarine, hot-pepper sauce, salt, black pepper, and tarragon. Cook for 5 minutes, or just until heated through. Remove and discard the bay leaf before serving.

Makes 4 servings

NUTRITION AT A GLANCE

Per serving: 210 calories, 8 g fat, 2 g saturated fat, 18 g protein, 18 g carbohydrate, 2 g dietary fiber, 45 mg cholesterol, 830 mg sodium

Lobster Bisque

Silky and full-flavored, bisques make any meal an elegant celebration. This easy version uses lobster tails to make preparation a breeze.

2 tablespoons canola oil

1 onion, finely chopped

2 tablespoons whole wheat flour

3 1/2 cups chicken broth

1/2 cup tomato puree

1/4 cup dry sherry

1/4 teaspoon salt

1 pound lobster tails, shells removed and cut into 1" pieces

1 1/4 cups 1% milk

1/4 teaspoon hot-pepper sauce

1 teaspoon paprika

1 plum tomato, chopped

2 tablespoons chopped parsley

Heat the oil in a large saucepan over medium-high heat. Add the onion and cook, stirring occasionally, for 5 minutes, or until tender. Stir in the flour and cook, stirring constantly, for 3 minutes, or until lightly browned.

Stir in the broth, tomato puree, sherry, and salt and bring to a boil. Reduce the heat to low, cover, and simmer for 10 minutes. Add the lobster, cover, and simmer for 6 minutes, or until the lobster is opaque.

Stir in the milk, hot-pepper sauce, and paprika. Cook over medium heat for 3 minutes, or until heated through. Stir in the plum tomatoes and parsley.

Makes 4 servings

NUTRITION AT A GLANCE

Per serving: 262 calories, 9 g fat, 1 g saturated fat, 27 g protein, 15 g carbohydrate, 2 g dietary fiber, 84 mg cholesterol, 742 mg sodium

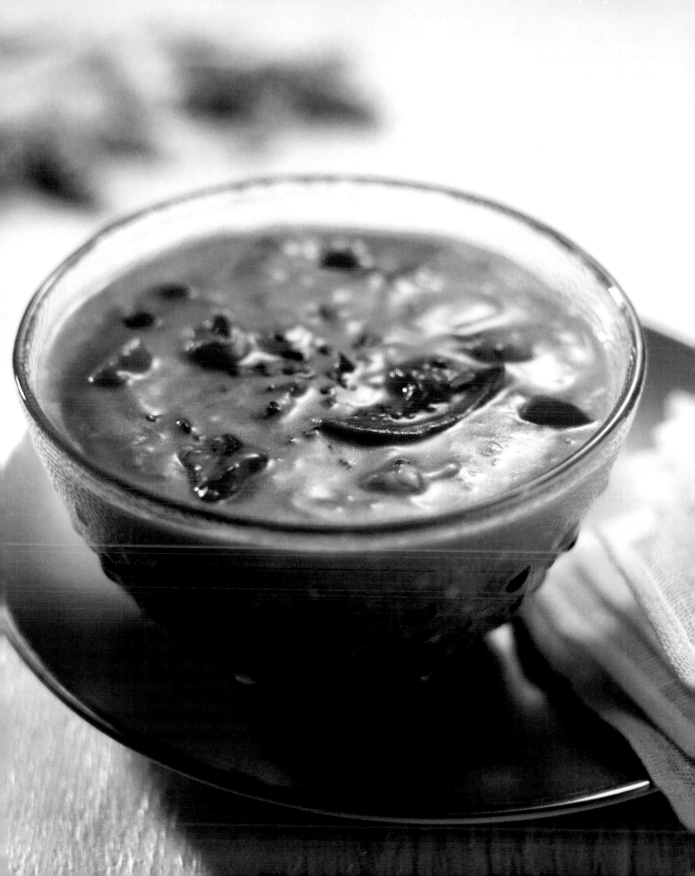

Chicken and Red Lentil Soup

To give this dish an Indian flair, you can add some shredded unsweetened coconut as an additional garnish.

1	tablespoon extra virgin olive oil
2	small carrots, finely chopped
2	large ribs celery, finely chopped
1/2	large onion, sliced
1 1/2	cloves garlic, minced
1	teaspoon curry powder
1/4	teaspoon ground ginger
1/4	teaspoon ground cumin
1/4	teaspoon hot red-pepper flakes
3/4	cup red lentils
2	pounds boneless, skinless chicken breasts
3	cups chicken broth
1 1/2	teaspoons tomato paste
2	cups water
	Sliced scallion, for garnish

Heat the oil in a large pot over medium heat. Add the carrots, celery, onion, garlic, curry powder, ginger, cumin, and pepper flakes. Cover and cook for 15 minutes, stirring occasionally until the vegetables have softened. Stir in the lentils and place the chicken on top. Add the broth.

In a cup, combine the tomato paste with a small amount of the water, then stir into the vegetable mixture. Add the remaining water. Partially cover and simmer for 30 minutes, or until the vegetables are soft and the chicken is cooked through.

Remove the pot from the heat. Remove the chicken from the pot, place on a cutting board, and cut into shreds.

In a blender or food processor, puree 2 cups of the soup, then return it to the pot, along with the shredded chicken.

Evenly divide the soup among 4 serving bowls. Sprinkle the scallion on top for garnish.

Makes 4 servings

NUTRITION AT A GLANCE
Per serving: 455 calories, 8 g fat, 2 g saturated fat, 64 g protein, 30 g carbohydrate, 8 g dietary fiber, 132 mg cholesterol, 972 mg sodium

Chicken and Veggie Chowder

Move over, chicken noodle! A puree of favorite vegetables thickens this sensational chowder. Serve this chowder with whole grain bread to make a hearty one-dish meal.

- 3 cups chicken broth
- 2 carrots, chopped
- 2 ribs celery, chopped
- 1 onion, chopped
- 2 ounces mushrooms, sliced
- 1 clove garlic, minced
- 1 teaspoon chopped fresh thyme leaves
- 1/4 teaspoon salt
- 1 pound boneless, skinless chicken breast, cut into 3/4" strips
- 2 tablespoons trans-free margarine
- 3 tablespoons whole wheat flour
- 1 cup 1% milk
- 3 spears asparagus, cut into 1" pieces, or 1 cup broccoli florets
- 1 tablespoon chopped parsley
- 1/4 teaspoon ground black pepper

In a large pot, combine the broth, carrots, celery, onion, mushrooms, garlic, thyme, and salt. Bring to a boil over high heat. Reduce the heat to low, cover, and simmer for 20 minutes, or until the vegetables are tender. Using a slotted spoon, remove half of the vegetable mixture to a food processor and process until pureed. Return to the saucepan.

Stir in the chicken, cover, and simmer for 15 minutes, or until the chicken is no longer pink.

Melt the margarine in a small saucepan over medium heat. Stir in the flour until smooth and cook for 1 minute. Gradually add the milk and cook, stirring constantly, for 3 minutes, or until thickened. Stir into the chicken mixture. Add the asparagus or broccoli, parsley, and pepper and cook for 5 minutes, or until heated through.

Makes 4 servings

NUTRITION AT A GLANCE

Per serving: 200 calories, 8 g fat, 2 g saturated fat, 13 g protein, 19 g carbohydrate, 4 g dietary fiber, 20 mg cholesterol, 1,058 mg sodium

Vegetable Beef Soup

Some soups are hearty; this soup is good for your heart because of all of the fiber from the cabbage, spinach, and celery.

2	tablespoons extra virgin olive oil
1	pound top round steak, trimmed and cut into 1 1/4" cubes
1	rib celery, finely chopped
1/2	large onion, finely chopped
1/4	pound green beans, cut into 1" pieces
5	cups water
1/4	small head cabbage, coarsely shredded
1/4	bag (from 10-ounce bag) spinach, coarsely shredded
1	can (16 ounce) diced tomatoes
	Ground black pepper

Heat 2 tablespoons of the oil in a large saucepan over medium-high heat. Add the steak and cook, stirring occasionally, for 8 minutes, or until well-browned on all sides and no longer pink in the center. Remove to a large bowl lined with paper towels. Cover the steak with a layer of paper towels.

Heat the remaining 2 tablespoons oil in the same saucepan over medium heat. Add the celery, onion, and green beans and cook, stirring occasionally, for 10 minutes, or until the vegetables are lightly browned.

Add the steak, water, cabbage, spinach, tomatoes (with juice), and pepper to taste. Bring to a boil over high heat, stirring frequently. Reduce the heat to low, cover, and simmer, stirring occasionally, for 1 1/2 hours, or until the steak is fork-tender.

Makes 4 servings

NUTRITION AT A GLANCE

Per serving: 290 calories, 17 g fat, 4 1/2 g saturated fat, 24 g protein, 11 g carbohydrate, 4 g dietary fiber, 60 mg cholesterol, 420 mg sodium

MY SOUTH BEACH DIET

I LOVE THE SIMPLICITY OF THIS PLAN.

I've become a walking advertisement for the South Beach Diet. I have lost 35 pounds in 3 months, and everyone who sees me wants to know how I've done it.

Three months ago, I weighed 190 pounds. At 43 years of age, with PCOS (Polycystic Ovary Syndrome) and a family history of heart disease and diabetes, I was afraid that I wouldn't be around to watch my two precious girls grow up. I weighed 110 pounds when I was first married, but years of struggling with infertility and two hard-won pregnancies took their toll.

In desperation, I started the Atkins diet even though I had misgivings about all the fat in that plan. Two days later, my mother called me from the Canyon Ranch health spa where, she said, the South Beach Diet was all the rage. I walked to the bookstore to buy the book and read it that night. The next day, I switched to the South Beach Diet, and I honestly feel like it is a change for life. Of the many things I love about it, foremost is its flexibility. I stuck pretty closely to Phase 1 for the first 2 weeks.

Since then, I have successfully gone on vacation, celebrated a birthday with a wonderful dinner that included dessert, and sampled several desserts prepared by one of the country's top French pastry chefs. Whenever I do treat myself or stray a bit, I always go back to a South Beach breakfast the next day, and I'm right back on track.

I think one of my greatest reasons for success with this plan is its simplicity. With two small children, it is important to me that there are no points to count, lists of foods to memorize, or special exercises that need to be done.

Right now my exercise is limited to pushing my 1 1/2-year-old daughter in a stroller or walking my older daughter to her gymnastics or ice skating classes, and I am still losing weight!

Also, as promised in the diet, I have not had any cravings since my second day on the diet, and I've never been hungry. I really do see this as the way that I will eat, and teach my family to eat, for the rest of my life. —*ELLEN S.*

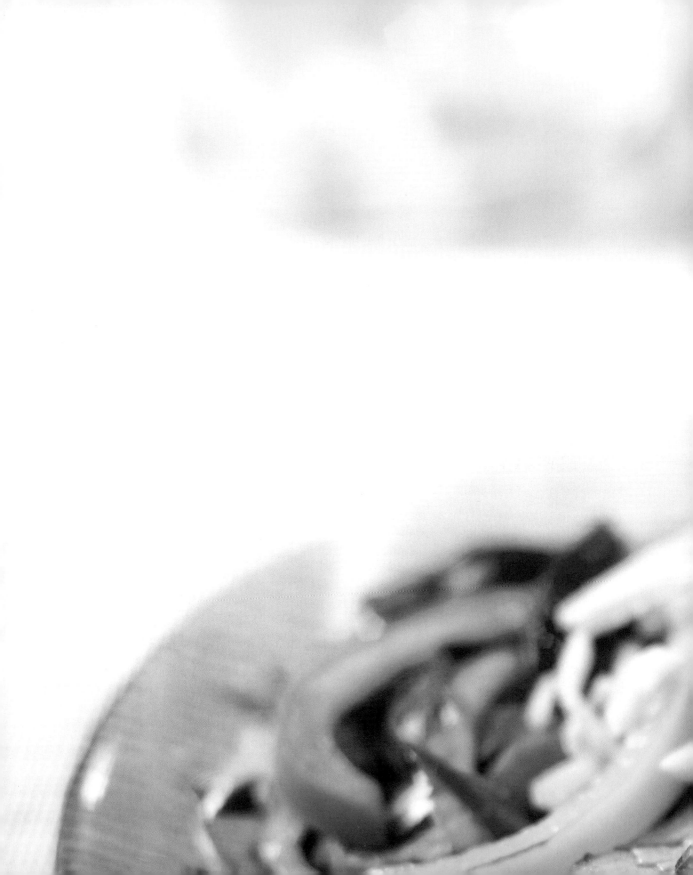

SALADS

For people trying to lose excess weight, there may be nothing more predictable—and less welcome—than suggestions for salads. Our goal was to come up with salads that contain enough protein—meat, fish, and cheese—to truly satisfy your hunger. Vegetarians can add beans instead of meat for bulk, flavor, and protein. Expand your idea of the vegetables in a salad to choose things that are healthier and more substantial than just lettuce or spinach. Salads are also a good way to use leftover meat or fish from the day before.

We steer clear of low-fat dressings, which usually contain sugars. Instead of low-fat, feel free to use a good vinaigrette or olive oil and vinegar dressing. Any mayonnaise-based dressing is also fine, since most mayo is just canola or olive oil, eggs, vinegar, and other flavorings. It's also easy today to find commercially made sugar-free dressings, such as those made by Walden Farms or Newman's Own.

Tropical Shrimp and Black Bean Salad

Colorful tropical fruits enhance this shrimp and black bean salad. It's terrific for lunch or a light dinner.

1	pound medium cooked shrimp, peeled and deveined
1	can (14–19 ounces) black beans, rinsed and drained
1	jicama, peeled and julienned (about 1 1/2 cups)
1	ripe papaya, peeled, halved, seeded, and chopped
2	kiwifruit, peeled and sliced
1/2	medium red onion, thinly sliced
1/2	cup chopped fresh cilantro leaves
1/4	cup extra virgin olive oil

On serving plates, arrange the shrimp, beans, jicama, papaya, kiwifruit, onion, and cilantro. Drizzle with the oil.

Makes 4 servings

NUTRITION AT A GLANCE

Per serving: 400 calories, 16 g fat, 2 g saturated fat, 31 g protein, 32 g carbohydrate, 10 g dietary fiber, 221 mg cholesterol, 567 mg sodium

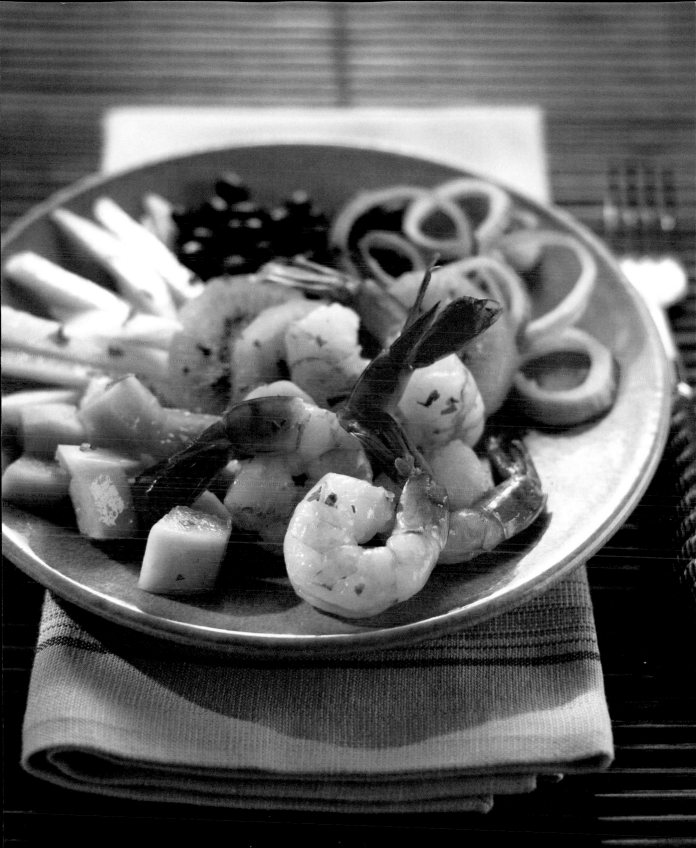

From the Menu of . . .

AZUL

Mandarin Oriental Hotel, 500 Brickell Key Drive, Miami

CHEF MICHELLE BERNSTEIN

AZUL IS A DRAMATIC DINING SPACE, WITH A WHITE MARBLE–CLAD OPEN KITCHEN AND PICTURESQUE BAY VIEWS FROM ITS FLOOR-TO-CEILING WINDOWS. AND THE FOOD IS AS SPECTACULAR AS THE VIEW.

Shaved Fennel Salad with Seared Tuna and Parmesan

PHASE 1

Salad

- 1 fennel bulb, shaved paper thin with a Japanese mandoline or meat slicer
- 2 tablespoons extra virgin olive oil
- 2 tablespoons fresh lemon juice
- 1/8 teaspoon chopped thyme leaves
- 1 teaspoon chopped Italian parsley
- 2 tablespoons shaved Reggiano or Parmesan cheese

Tuna

1/4	teaspoon salt
1	tablespoon pink peppercorns
4	ounces tuna (fresh sushi grade)
1 1/2	teaspoon extra virgin olive oil

To make the salad: Mix the fennel, oil, lemon juice, thyme, Italian parsley, and cheese. Set aside in a cool place.

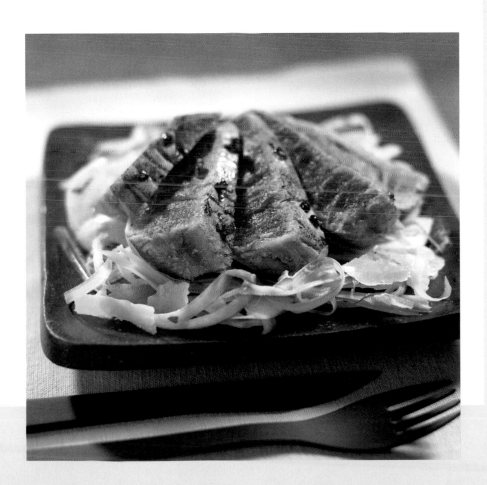

To make the tuna: Sprinkle the salt and peppercorns on the tuna. Place a sauté pan on high heat and add the olive oil. Place the tuna in the pan and allow to cook 30 seconds or 1 minute on each side. Remove from the pan and slice into 5 pieces.

Place the fennel salad on a flat plate and place the slices of tuna in the center of the salad. Serve immediately.

Makes 1 serving

NUTRITION AT A GLANCE

Per serving: 460 calories, 27 g fat, 6 g saturated fat, 36 g protein, 22 g carbohydrate, 9 g dietary fiber, 65 mg cholesterol, 910 mg sodium

Tuna and Bean Salad

With the saltiness of the capers and the smoothness of the sour cream and mayonnaise, this tuna salad really comes to life. Enjoy it for a satisfying lunch.

2	bunches watercress, tough ends trimmed
1/4	cup water
1	clove garlic, thinly sliced
1	can (12 ounces) tuna, packed in water, drained and flaked
1/2	cup rinsed and drained canned cannellini beans
1/4	sweet white onion, finely chopped
1/2	cup chopped roasted red pepper
3	tablespoons mayonnaise
2	tablespoons fat-free sour cream
1	tablespoon red wine vinegar
1 1/2	teaspoons rinsed and drained capers
	Salt
	Ground black pepper

Coarsely chop the watercress stems until you have 1/2 cup. Rinse and dry the remaining watercress sprigs and set aside.

In a small saucepan, combine the chopped stems, water, and garlic. Bring to a boil over medium-high heat. Reduce the heat to low. Cover and simmer until the watercress stems are bright green, about 1 to 2 minutes. Drain and place in a large bowl. Add the tuna, beans, onion, and roasted pepper to the bowl and toss to blend.

In a blender or food processor, combine the mayonnaise, sour cream, vinegar, capers, and salt and black pepper to taste. Puree until smooth.

Serve the tuna mixture on the reserved watercress sprigs. Drizzle with the dressing.

Makes 4 servings

NUTRITION AT A GLANCE

Per serving: 222 calories, 11 g fat, 2 g saturated fat, 23 g protein, 8 g carbohydrate, 2 g dietary fiber, 40 mg cholesterol, 543 mg sodium

Asian Chicken Salad with Wonton Crisps

You'll love the sweet-and-sour taste of this crunchy chicken salad. Wonton wrappers and traditional ingredients provide authentic Asian flare.

8	wonton wrappers, cut into 1/4" strips
1/4	cup rice vinegar or white wine vinegar
2	tablespoons hoisin sauce
2	tablespoons canola oil
1/4	teaspoon sesame oil
1	tablespoon grated fresh ginger
1	clove garlic, minced
1/4	teaspoon crushed red-pepper flakes
1	pound mixed greens
1	cup bean sprouts
1/2	pound cooked shredded chicken breast
1	carrot, shredded
2	scallions, thinly sliced

Preheat the oven to 400°F. Coat a baking sheet with cooking spray.

Separate the wonton strips and place them on the prepared baking sheet. Coat them lightly with cooking spray. Bake for 3 minutes, or until golden brown and crisp. Remove and set aside.

In a large bowl, whisk together the vinegar, hoisin sauce, canola oil, sesame oil, ginger, garlic, and red–

pepper flakes until blended. Add the greens, sprouts, chicken, carrot, scallions, and reserved wonton strips. Toss gently to mix and serve immediately.

Makes 4 servings

NUTRITION AT A GLANCE

Per serving: 274 calories, 10 g fat, 1 g saturated fat, 23 g protein, 23 g carbohydrate, 5 g dietary fiber, 50 mg cholesterol, 498 mg sodium

Smoked Chicken Salad with Raspberry-Balsamic Vinaigrette

If you need a meal in minutes, this is just what you're looking for. This can also be eaten as a dinner salad in the summer when you just don't want to turn on the oven.

1/4	cup sugar-free raspberry jam
3	tablespoons extra virgin olive oil
1/4	cup balsamic vinegar
3/4	pound boneless smoked chicken breast, cut into 3" strips
6	cups mesclun mix
2	cups fresh raspberries
1/4	cup toasted sliced almonds

In a resealable jar, combine the jam, oil, and vinegar. Close the lid tightly and shake vigorously.

In a large bowl, gently toss the chicken with the dressing. Line a large platter or bowl with the mesclun. Top with the chicken mixture, raspberries, and almonds. (Or, if desired, place the chicken on the mesclun and serve the dressing on the side or drizzled over the top and topped with the raspberries and almonds.)

Makes 4 servings

Per serving: 275 calories, 17 g fat, 3 g saturated fat, 18 g protein, 25 g carbohydrate, 6 g dietary fiber, 33 mg cholesterol, 800 mg sodium

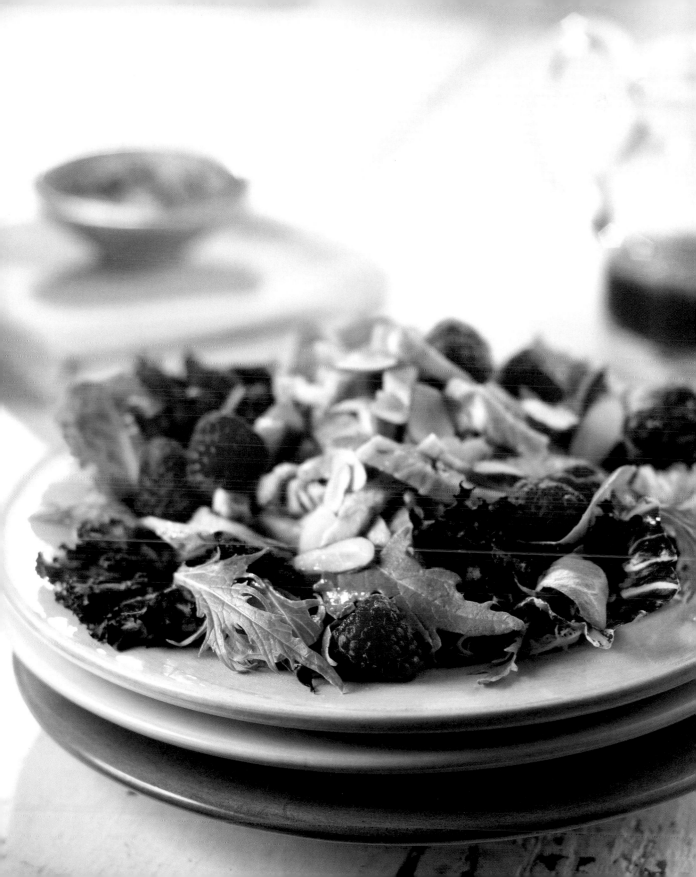

Chicken Salad

This salad is so simple to make, you'll have no reason to fear preparing it, or serving it anytime.

3/4 cup fat-free sour cream

3 scallions, minced

1 tablespoon finely chopped parsley

1/2 teaspoon grated lemon peel

Salt

Ground black pepper

3 cups shredded cooked chicken breast

8 large leaves lettuce

In a medium bowl, combine the sour cream, scallions, parsley, lemon peel, and salt and pepper to taste. Toss well to blend. Add the chicken and toss to coat. Serve on a bed of lettuce leaves.

Makes 4 servings

NUTRITION AT A GLANCE

Per serving: 234 calories, 5 g fat, 1 g saturated fat, 35 g protein, 11 g carbohydrate, 2 g dietary fiber, 94 mg cholesterol, 127 mg sodium

Frisée Salad with Blue Cheese and Walnuts

A fruity vinaigrette with a Dijon tang is the perfect topping for this salad. The sprinkling of walnuts and blue cheese takes it over the top.

Raspberry Vinaigrette

    1 tablespoon sugar-free raspberry fruit spread
    1/2 cup balsamic vinegar
    1 1/2 teaspoons walnut or canola oil
    1/2 teaspoon Dijon mustard

Salad

    1/4 cup dry red wine
    1 pear, cored and chopped
    4 cups mixed frisée or baby lettuce
    2 tablespoons toasted walnuts, chopped
    2 tablespoons crumbled blue cheese
    Salt
    Ground black pepper

To make the raspberry vinaigrette: Place the fruit spread in a small microwaveable bowl and microwave on high power for 1 minute, or until melted. Whisk in the vinegar, oil, and mustard.

To make the salad: Combine the wine and pear in a small saucepan over medium-high heat. Cook, stirring often, for 4 minutes, or until the liquid has evaporated.

Divide the frisée or lettuce among 4 dinner plates. Sprinkle with the walnuts and blue cheese. Sprinkle with salt and pepper to taste. Divide the pear among the plates. Drizzle with vinaigrette.

Makes 4 servings

NUTRITION AT A GLANCE
Per serving: 130 calories, 5 g fat, 1 g saturated fat, 2 g protein, 18 g carbohydrate, 3 g dietary fiber, 5 mg cholesterol, 160 mg sodium

Chinese Beef and Pepper Salad

Whether you're making this from scratch or using yesterday's leftover London broil, the results will be equally satisfying.

1/3 cup light soy sauce

2 tablespoons extra virgin olive oil

1 tablespoon dry sherry

2 teaspoons sugar substitute

1 teaspoon ground ginger

1 small clove garlic, minced

1 pound cooked London broil, trimmed of all visible fat and cut into slivers about 1/8" wide and 1" long

1 medium red bell pepper, cut into very thin slivers

2 scallions, sliced

In a small bowl whisk together the soy sauce, oil, sherry, sugar substitute, ginger, and garlic. Add the beef and toss to coat. Cover and refrigerate for up to 1 day, until ready to use.

Drain the beef and reserve the marinade. Place the beef on a serving plate and toss with the pepper and scallions. Serve with the reserved marinade on the side.

Makes 4 servings

NUTRITION AT A GLANCE

Per serving: 283 calories, 15 g fat, 5 g saturated fat, 24 g protein, 9 g carbohydrate, 2 g dietary fiber, 54 mg cholesterol, 860 mg sodium

Tiered Salad with Lime Dressing

If you're looking for a cool, refreshing lunch this summer, you've found it. Make this the night before, keep it in the refrigerator, and when you're ready, it's ready.

Lime Dressing

- 1/3 cup lime juice
- 1/4 cup chopped fresh cilantro
- 1 scallion, chopped
- 1 tablespoon extra virgin olive oil
- 1 teaspoon sugar substitute
- 1/2 teaspoon salt
- 3 medium avocados, peeled and pitted
- 1/2 cup picante sauce
- 2 tablespoons lemon juice

Tiered Salad

- 1 cup cherry tomatoes, halved
- 1 cup mixed greens
- 1 large yellow bell pepper, chopped
- 1 1/2 cups cauliflower florets
- 1 cup chopped cooked turkey ham
- 1/2 cup cooked or canned chickpeas
- 1/4 cup sliced black olives
- Finely chopped yellow bell pepper, for garnish

To make the lime dressing: In a small bowl, combine the lime juice, cilantro, scallion, oil, sugar substitute, and salt. Add the avocados and mash to incorporate. Stir in the picante sauce and lemon juice.

To make the tiered salad: In a 2-quart glass salad bowl, arrange the tomatoes, cut sides down. Place the greens over the tomatoes. Top with the bell pepper, then the cauliflower, turkey ham, and chickpeas. Top with half of the lime dressing. Top the dish with the olives. Serve with the remaining dressing on the side. Garnish with the yellow bell pepper.

Makes 4 servings

NUTRITION AT A GLANCE
Per serving: 380 calories, 27 g fat, 5 g saturated fat, 12 g protein, 28 g carbohydrate, 15 g dietary fiber, 20 mg cholesterol, 1,170 mg sodium

Pork and Pepper Salad with Balsamic Vinaigrette

When you're in a real hurry, use leftover pork (or chicken) and jarred roasted peppers instead of starting with fresh. Just warm them in the microwave.

 1 red bell pepper

 1 green bell pepper

 1 yellow bell pepper

 1/2 pound lean pork tenderloin

 1 tablespoon extra virgin olive oil

 1 medium red onion, thinly sliced

 2 cups red or green cabbage, thinly sliced

 2 ribs celery, thinly sliced

 1/2 teaspoon salt

 1/8 teaspoon ground black pepper

 1/4 cup sugar-free balsamic vinaigrette dressing

 1/4 cup (1 ounce) shredded reduced-fat Muenster or mozzarella cheese

Preheat the broiler. Place the bell peppers on a broiler pan and cook 4" from the heat, turning occasionally, until the skin is bubbly and browned all over. Place in a paper bag, seal, and set aside for 5 minutes, or until cool enough to handle. Remove, halve, and discard the skin, ribs, and seeds. Cut the peppers into strips.

Place the pork on the broiler pan and cook for 12 minutes, turning once, or until a thermometer inserted

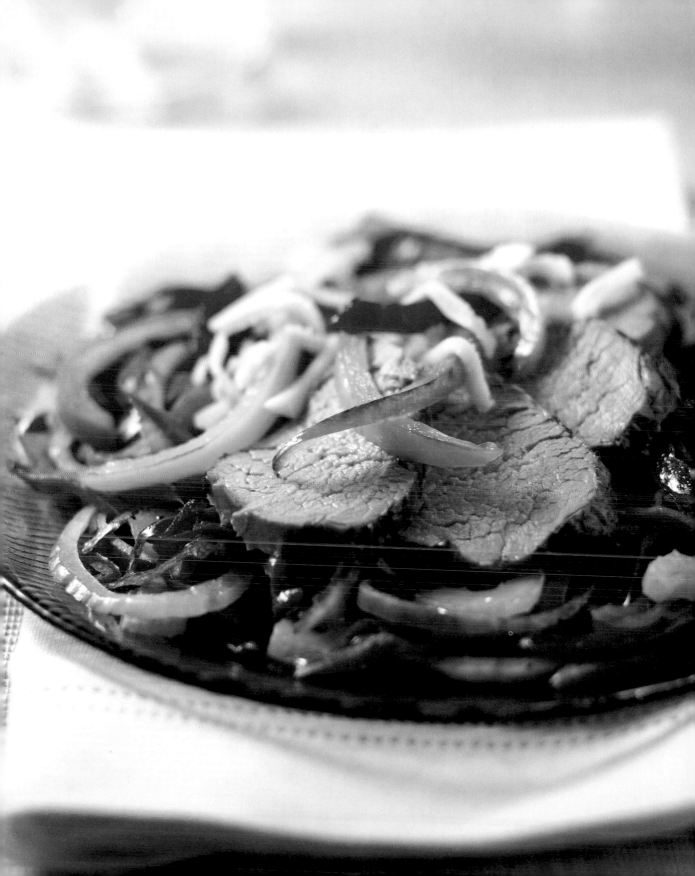

in center reaches 155°F and the juices run clear. Let stand for 10 minutes before cutting into thin slices.

Warm the oil in a medium skillet over medium heat. Add the onion, cabbage, celery, salt, and black pepper. Cook, stirring frequently, for 10 minutes, or until tender.

Divide the cabbage mixture among 4 plates. Arrange the peppers and pork on top. Drizzle each with dressing and sprinkle with 1 tablespoon cheese.

Makes 4 servings

NUTRITION AT A GLANCE
Per serving: 194 calories, 8 g fat, 2 g saturated fat, 16 g protein, 16 g carbohydrate, 4 g dietary fiber, 43 mg cholesterol, 631 mg sodium

Mixed Greens with Creamy Poppy Seed Dressing

Poppy seed dressing is a delightfully sweet and nutty way to top a salad. To enhance the seeds' flavor even more, lightly toast them in a dry skillet for 2 to 3 minutes before adding them to the dressing.

Dressing

- 1/2 cup fat-free plain yogurt
- 2 tablespoons orange juice
- 2 teaspoons poppy seeds
- 1/2 teaspoon apple cider vinegar
- Pinch of ground black pepper

Salad

- 1 head red leaf lettuce, coarsely torn
- 1 bunch watercress
- 1 cup cherry tomato halves

To make the dressing: In a small bowl, whisk together the yogurt, orange juice, poppy seeds, vinegar, and pepper.

To make the salad: In a salad bowl, combine the lettuce, watercress, and tomatoes. Add the dressing and toss gently.

Makes 4 servings

NUTRITION AT A GLANCE

Per serving: 49 calories, 1 g fat, 0 g saturated fat, 4 g protein, 9 g carbohydrate, 2 g dietary fiber, 1 mg cholesterol, 39 mg sodium

CHEF JONATHAN EISMANN

PACIFIC TIME IS A WELL-KNOWN PAN-ASIAN EATERY ON MIAMI'S CAR-FREE LINCOLN ROAD. WINDOW SHOPPING AT NEIGHBORING BOUTIQUES AND GALLERIES IS A FAVORITE PRE- OR POST-DINNER ACTIVITY.

Vegetable (Chinese Long Bean) Salad with Feta

PHASE 1

Dressing

1/4	cup Chinese black vinegar
2	tablespoons strong brewed dark tea
2	tablespoons lime juice
2	tablespoons finely chopped chives
2	tablespoons finely chopped lemongrass

Vegetable Salad

1/2	pound Chinese long beans or green beans cut into 1/2 " pieces

1	cup crumbled feta cheese
1	cup mung bean sprouts
1/4	cup finely chopped scallions, green parts only
1	medium cucumber, peeled, seeded, and cut into 1/4" cubes
1	red bell pepper, julienned
	Salt
	Ground white pepper

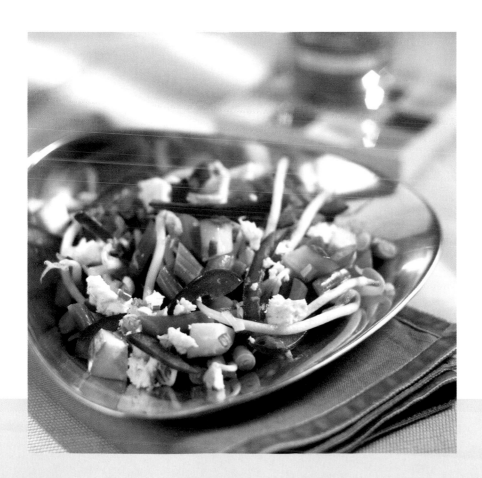

To make the dressing: In a medium bowl, combine the vinegar, tea, lime juice, chives, and lemongrass.

To make the salad: Blanch the beans in boiling water for about 2 minutes.

In a large bowl, combine the beans with the cheese, bean sprouts, scallions, cucumber, and bell pepper. Mix with the dressing. Adjust seasoning to taste with salt and ground white pepper.

Chill before serving.

Makes 4 servings

NUTRITION AT A GLANCE

Per serving: 137 calories, 4 g fat, 3 g saturated fat, 11 g protein, 15 g carbohydrate, 4 g dietary fiber, 13 mg cholesterol, 493 mg sodium

Green Bean and Red Onion Salad

A quick onion sauté makes a colorful splash over fresh green beans and cucumber. You can reduce the amount of garlic if you prefer a slightly milder taste.

2 pounds green beans, steamed and chilled

1 cucumber, seeded and julienned

2 red onions, sliced and separated into rings

3 cloves garlic, minced

3 tablespoons extra virgin olive oil

1/4 cup red wine vinegar

2 tablespoons water

1 teaspoon sugar substitute

In a large bowl, combine the beans and cucumber.

In a small skillet, sauté the onion and garlic in 2 tablespoons of the oil until tender but not browned. Stir in the vinegar, water, and sugar substitute and simmer for 2 minutes, stirring until the sugar substitute is dissolved. Stir in the remaining oil. Spoon the onion dressing over the bean mixture. Serve immediately.

Makes 6 servings

NUTRITION AT A GLANCE
Per serving: 138 calories, 6 g fat, 0 g saturated fat, 4 g protein, 16 g carbohydrate, 6 g dietary fiber, 0 mg cholesterol, 2 mg sodium

Sesame Snow Pea and Asparagus Salad

Snow peas and sesame are a natural combination. Adding fresh asparagus makes for a very elegant and classy salad. Serve this alongside a main dish, or enjoy it as a light lunch.

1 1/2 cups cooked brown rice
2 tablespoons canola oil
2 teaspoons sesame oil
3 tablespoons light soy sauce
1/2 pound snow peas, trimmed and cooked
1/2 pound fresh asparagus, trimmed and cooked
3 tablespoons sesame seeds, toasted
3 scallions, sliced
1/4 teaspoon crushed red-pepper flakes

In a large serving bowl, toss the rice with the canola oil, sesame oil, and soy sauce. Stir in the snow peas, asparagus, and sesame seeds and toss to combine. Sprinkle with the scallions and red-pepper flakes.

Makes 6 servings

NUTRITION AT A GLANCE
Per serving: 239 calories, 9 g fat, 1 g saturated fat, 6 g protein, 31 g carbohydrate, 5 g dietary fiber, 0 mg cholesterol, 314 mg sodium

Fava Beans and Greens

Fava beans are also called by many other names, including broad beans and horse beans. Whatever they are called, they contain more protein than chickpeas, kidney beans, pintos, lentils, limas, or peas and just a tenth of the fat of soybeans.

2 cups arugula

2 cups mixed greens

1 can (14–19 ounces) fava beans, rinsed and drained

1/4 red onion, thinly sliced

South Beach Green Goddess Dressing (see page 235)

In a large bowl, combine the arugula, greens, beans, and onion and toss thoroughly. Serve with South Beach Green Goddess dressing.

Makes 4 servings

NUTRITION AT A GLANCE

Per serving: 91 calories, 1 g fat, 0 g saturated fat, 5 g protein, 16 g carbohydrate, 5 g dietary fiber, 0 mg cholesterol, 229 mg sodium

Artichoke Salad with Olives

Wake up your taste buds with this break from the traditional green salad. Using frozen artichoke hearts and jarred roasted bell pepper helps streamline the prep time, so you can have the salad ready in a snap.

1/4	cup mayonnaise
2	tablespoons sugar-free creamy Italian dressing
1/8	teaspoon ground black pepper
1	package (10 ounces) frozen artichoke hearts, thawed and chopped
1/2	cup chopped roasted red bell pepper
1	rib celery, chopped
1/4	cup chopped fresh basil
8	kalamata olives, pitted and halved
6	leaves lettuce

In a small bowl, whisk together the mayonnaise, Italian dressing, and black pepper.

In a large serving bowl, combine the artichokes, roasted pepper, celery, basil, and olives. Stir in the dressing. Cover and refrigerate until ready to serve.

Divide the lettuce among six plates. Spoon the artichoke mixture onto the lettuce.

Makes 6 servings

NUTRITION AT A GLANCE

Per serving: 120 calories, 11 g fat, 1 1/2 g saturated fat, 2 g protein, 6 g carbohydrate, 3 g dietary fiber, 5 mg cholesterol, 250 mg sodium

Vegetable Salad

Green runs supreme in this tasty lunch. This salad is also delicious topped with cold chicken or shrimp.

1/2 cup cut fresh green beans (cut into 1" lengths)

1/2 carrot, julienned

1/2 cup chopped fresh asparagus

1/4 cup frozen peas

1/2 cup torn spinach

1/2 small bulb fennel, thinly sliced

1/2 tomato, chopped

1/2 cup white mushrooms, sliced

1/2 cup curly endive, shredded

1/2 small summer squash, sliced

1/4 cucumber, thinly sliced

1/4 cup sliced radishes

Herbed Vinaigrette, as desired (see recipe on page 238)

Belgian endive leaves

Chopped fresh cilantro, for garnish

Heat a small amount of water in a small saucepan over medium heat. Add the green beans and gently boil for 4 to 6 minutes. Add the carrot. Cook for 2 minutes. Add the asparagus and peas. Cook for 2 minutes. Drain well and rinse with cold water. Drain again.

In a large salad bowl, combine the spinach, fennel, tomato, mushrooms, curly endive, squash, cucumber, and radishes. Add the cooked vegetables and the Herbed Vinaigrette. Toss well to coat all the vegetables.

To serve, line a platter with the Belgian endive, then spoon the vegetables on top. Sprinkle the cilantro over the top for garnish.

Makes 4 servings

NUTRITION AT A GLANCE

Per serving: 44 calories, 0 g fat, 0 g saturated fat, 3 g protein, 9 g carbohydrate, 4 g dietary fiber, 0 mg cholesterol, 44 mg sodium

Balsamic Tomato and Mozzarella Salad

Tomato and fresh basil are a classic combination in Italian cuisine. If you don't have time to roast fresh peppers, you can use jarred roasted peppers instead.

1	tablespoon balsamic vinegar
1	teaspoon extra virgin olive oil
1	teaspoon flaxseed oil
1	clove garlic, minced
1/4	teaspoon salt
1/8	teaspoon ground black pepper
2	large red bell peppers, halved and seeded
2	large tomatoes, cut into 1/2"-thick slices
2	ounces fresh mozzarella cheese, cut into 4 slices
1/3	cup fresh basil leaves, julienned

Preheat the broiler. Coat a broiler-pan rack with cooking spray.

In a cup, whisk together the vinegar, olive oil, flaxseed oil, garlic, salt, and black pepper. Set aside.

Place the bell peppers, skin side up, on the prepared rack. Broil, without turning, for 10 minutes, or until the skins are blackened and blistered in spots.

Place the peppers in a paper bag and seal. Let stand for 10 minutes, or until cool enough to handle. Peel the skin from the peppers and discard. Cut the peppers into 1/2 "-wide strips.

Arrange the tomato slices on a platter. Place the cheese slices over the tomatoes. Scatter the pepper strips on top and sprinkle with the basil. Drizzle the dressing over the salad. Let stand for at least 15 minutes to allow the flavors to blend.

Makes 4 servings

NUTRITION AT A GLANCE

Per serving: 100 calories, 5 g fat, 2 g saturated fat, 5 g protein, 9 g carbohydrate, 2 g dietary fiber, 8 mg cholesterol, 241 mg sodium

Sweet Potato Salad

Here's a healthy alternative to traditional potato salad. Try serving at your next backyard picnic.

1 1/2	pounds sweet potatoes, scrubbed
1	large apple, peeled, cored, and cubed
1	large rib celery, chopped
1	tablespoon orange juice
1	tablespoon extra virgin olive oil
2	teaspoons apple cider vinegar
1	teaspoon sugar substitute
	Pinch of salt

Place the sweet potatoes in a large saucepan and cover with water. Bring to a boil over medium heat and cook for 30 minutes, or until tender. Drain and cool. Peel and cut into cubes.

In a large bowl, combine the sweet potatoes, apple, and celery.

In a small bowl, whisk together the orange juice, oil, vinegar, sugar substitute, and salt. Pour the mixture over the potato mixture and toss to coat. Cover and refrigerate until ready to serve.

Makes 4 servings

NUTRITION AT A GLANCE

Per serving: 248 calories, 4 g fat, 1 g saturated fat, 3 g protein, 51 g carbohydrate, 7 g dietary fiber, 0 mg cholesterol, 35 mg sodium

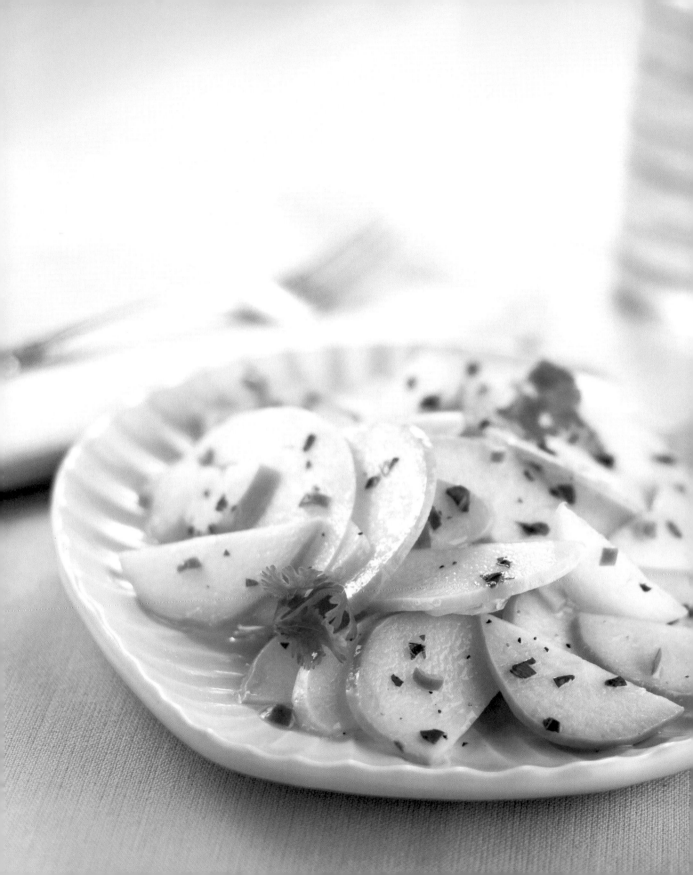

Chayote Salad

The chayote was a favorite fruit of the Aztecs and Mayans. It's also known as vegetable pear, mirliton, and christophene. When you go shopping for chayote, remember that they age much as we do, so if they're wrinkled, they're old. When young, the chayote skin is tender and quite edible. If your selection is not as young as you'd prefer, peel away the skin before you slice it.

  3 chayote, pitted and thinly sliced
  1 serrano chile pepper, seeded and finely chopped (wear plastic gloves when handling)
1/4 cup chopped fresh cilantro
     Juice of 1 small lemon, strained
1/3 cup extra virgin olive oil
  2 tablespoons apple cider vinegar
     Salt
     Freshly ground black pepper
     Small sprigs cilantro, for garnish

In a large bowl, combine the chayote, chile pepper, cilantro, lemon juice, oil, and vinegar. Toss to coat well. Sprinkle with salt and pepper. Garnish with the cilantro sprigs.

Makes 4 servings

NUTRITION AT A GLANCE

Per serving: 222 calories, 18 g fat, 4 g saturated fat, 1 g protein, 7 g carbohydrate, 3 g dietary fiber, 0 mg cholesterol, 6 mg sodium

Couscous Salad

This light salad is a perfect summer side dish.

- 1/2 cup couscous
- 1 teaspoon chicken bouillon granules
- 1 cup boiling water
- 1 medium tomato, seeded and finely chopped
- 1 small cucumber, peeled and finely chopped
- 1/4 cup sugar-free balsamic vinaigrette dressing
- 1 bag (10 ounces) baby spinach leaves, stems removed
- 3 ounces crumbled reduced-fat feta cheese

In a large bowl, combine the couscous and bouillon granules. Stir in the water. Cover and set aside for 5 minutes, or until the liquid is absorbed. Add the tomato, cucumber, and dressing and toss until blended. Cover and refrigerate until ready to serve.

Just before serving, add 3 cups of spinach and the cheese to the couscous and toss. Line a serving platter with the remaining spinach leaves and spoon the couscous mixture over the top.

Makes 4 servings

NUTRITION AT A GLANCE

Per serving: 170 calories, 3 1/2 g fat, 1 1/2 g saturated fat, 9 g protein, 28 g carbohydrate, 5 g dietary fiber, 10 mg cholesterol, 680 mg sodium

Overnight Slaw

If you're looking for a delicious way to eat more fiber, it's hard to beat an old-fashioned slaw.

- 1/4–1/2 cup sugar substitute
- 1/4 cup lemon juice
- 1/4 cup white vinegar
- 1 teaspoon celery salt
- 1 teaspoon garlic salt
- 1 small head cabbage, shredded
- 3 ribs celery, chopped
- 1/2 green bell pepper, chopped
- 1/4 cup chopped fresh chives
- 1/4 cup sliced radishes

In a large bowl, whisk together the sugar substitute, lemon juice, vinegar, celery salt, and garlic salt. Add the cabbage, celery, green pepper, and chives and toss lightly. Cover and refrigerate overnight. Add the radishes immediately before serving.

Makes 4 servings

NUTRITION AT A GLANCE

Per serving: 106 calories, 1 g fat, 0 g saturated fat, 4 g protein, 25 g carbohydrate, 5 g dietary fiber, 0 mg cholesterol, 685 mg sodium

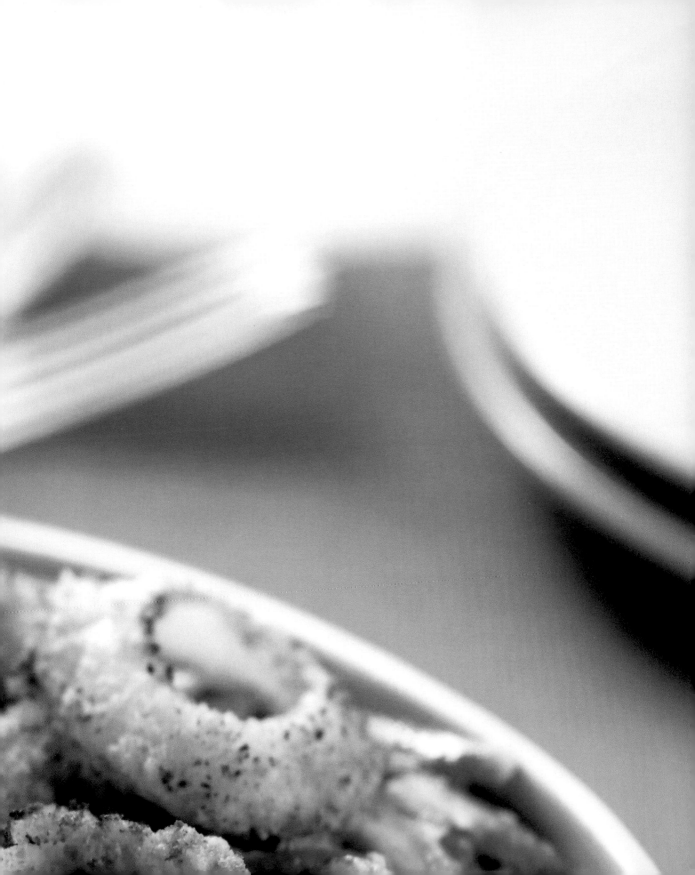

SIDE DISHES AND ACCOMPANIMENTS

The universe of side dishes can be divided into two main groups: the absolutely healthy kind (vegetables, for the most part, especially green ones) and the kind that supply starches and carbs such as potatoes, rice, noodles, dumplings, and the rest. Ideally, people on the South Beach Diet will rely heavily on the healthy vegetables. To assist in that effort, we've devised some new, tasty ways to prepare them, methods that turn out delicious and memorable dishes without adding any unnecessary starches.

In this chapter, you'll find recipes for Sesame-Ginger Asparagus, Summer Squash with Asiago Cheese—even a traditional Green Bean Casserole that's been slimmed down, South Beach style. There are also recipes for perfectly legal sauces and condiments.

Edamame with Scallions and Sesame

Edamame is the Japanese name for green soybeans. These tasty beans have exploded in popularity in recent years. Give them a try, and soon you'll be hooked! The easy cooking method used here has this dish ready in 15 minutes.

>   1 bag (12 ounces) frozen shelled edamame
>   1 tablespoon light soy sauce
>   1/2 cup water
> 1 1/2 teaspoons sesame oil
>   1 teaspoon canola oil
>   Dash of hot-pepper sauce (optional)
>   2 tablespoons finely chopped scallions
>   1/8 teaspoon ground black pepper

Bring the edamame, soy sauce, and water to a boil in a medium saucepan over medium-high heat. Reduce the heat to low and simmer, stirring occasionally, for 12 minutes, or until tender. If any liquid remains, cook, stirring occasionally, until the liquid has evaporated.

Remove from the heat. Stir in the sesame oil, canola oil, hot-pepper sauce, if using, scallions, and black pepper.

Makes 4 servings

NUTRITION AT A GLANCE

Per serving: 140 calories, 6 g fat, 0 g saturated fat, 10 g protein, 11 g carbohydrate, 5 g dietary fiber, 0 mg cholesterol, 430 mg sodium

Glazed Bell Peppers and Snow Peas

A sweet and tangy glaze of balsamic vinegar replaces butter in this spring side dish. If you prefer sugar snap peas, they work nicely in place of the snow peas.

    3 cups snow peas, trimmed
    2 tablespoons water
  1/3 cup balsamic vinegar
    1 teaspoon sugar substitute
    1 teaspoon extra virgin olive oil
  1/2 large red bell pepper, cut into short strips
    1 clove garlic, minced
  1/8 tablespoon salt
  1/8 teaspoon ground black pepper

Place the snow peas and water in a large microwaveable bowl. Cover with vented plastic wrap and microwave on high power for a total of 5 minutes, or until crisp-tender; stop and stir after 3 minutes. Drain.

Bring the vinegar and sugar substitute to a boil in a small saucepan over medium-high heat. Cook, stirring constantly, for 3 minutes, or until the mixture is reduced to 2 tablespoons. Remove from the heat.

Warm the oil in a large nonstick skillet over medium heat. Add the bell pepper and garlic and cook for 2 minutes, or until crisp-tender. Add the snow peas, salt, black pepper, and the vinegar glaze. Toss to mix.

Makes 4 servings

NUTRITION AT A GLANCE

Per serving: 45 calories, 0 g fat, 0 g saturated fat, 2 g protein, 9 g carbohydrate, 2 g dietary fiber, 0 mg cholesterol, 80 mg sodium

Sautéed Peppers and Onions

There's nothing quite so flavorful as sautéed peppers and onions, a tender-sweet combination that goes well with just about any main dish. Here the flavor is enhanced with the addition of full-bodied balsamic vinegar, along with some juicy tomatoes.

- 1 tablespoon extra virgin olive oil
- 4 large bell peppers, cut into 2" wedges
- 1 large red onion, sliced and separated into rings
- 1 tablespoon balsamic vinegar
- 1 teaspoon dried basil
- 1/4 teaspoon salt
- 1/4 teaspoon ground black pepper
- 2 plum tomatoes, chopped
- 3 tablespoons chicken or vegetable broth or water

Heat the oil in a large skillet over medium heat. Add the bell peppers and onion and cook, stirring occasionally, for 5 minutes, or until the onion starts to soften.

Add the vinegar, basil, salt, and black pepper and cook for 1 minute. Add the tomatoes and broth or water. Reduce the heat to low, cover, and simmer, stirring occasionally, for 8 minutes, or until the vegetables are very tender.

Makes 4 servings

NUTRITION AT A GLANCE

Per serving: 80 calories, 4 1/2 g fat, 1/2 g saturated fat, 2 g protein, 11 g carbohydrate, 4 g dietary fiber, 0 mg cholesterol, 210 mg sodium

Orange-Ginger Green Beans

Orange and ginger give ordinary green beans a snappy flavor from the Orient.

1 pound green beans
1 tablespoon trans-free margarine
1/2 cup chopped shallots
1 tablespoon finely chopped fresh ginger
1/2 teaspoon grated orange peel

Bring a medium saucepan of water to a boil over medium-high heat. Add the beans, cover, and simmer for 5 minutes, or until tender. Drain and remove to a bowl.

Melt the margarine in the same pan over low heat. Add the shallots and ginger and sauté for 5 minutes, or until the shallots are tender. Add the beans and orange peel and toss to combine.

Makes 8 servings

NUTRITION AT A GLANCE

Per serving: 35 calories, 1 g fat, 0 g saturated fat, 1 g protein, 5 g carbohydrate, 2 g dietary fiber, 0 mg cholesterol, 15 mg sodium

Homestyle Green Bean Casserole

No buffet or family gathering is complete without a green bean casserole. Here we've given this old favorite a South Beach update, so you can enjoy it in Phase 2 and beyond. Be prepared for lots of requests for this recipe!

- 1/2 cup buttermilk
- 1/4 cup whole wheat bread crumbs
- 1/4 cup ground walnuts
- 1 onion, cut crosswise into ¼-inch-thick slices and separated into rings
- 1/2 pound baby bella or cremini mushrooms, sliced
- 1 onion, chopped
- 1/2 teaspoon dried thyme
- 1/4 teaspoon salt
- 1/4 cup whole wheat flour
- 3 cups 1% milk
- 1 bag (16 ounces) frozen French-cut green beans, thawed and drained

Preheat the oven to 500°F. Coat a medium baking sheet and 13" × 9" baking dish with cooking spray.

Place the buttermilk in a shallow bowl. Place the bread crumbs and walnuts in another shallow bowl; stir to combine. Dip the onion rings into the buttermilk, then dredge in the bread crumbs and place on the prepared baking sheet. Coat the onion rings lightly with cooking spray.

Bake for 20 minutes, or until tender and golden brown.

Meanwhile, heat a medium saucepan coated with cooking spray over medium heat. Add the mushrooms, chopped onion, thyme, and salt. Coat with cooking spray. Cook, stirring occasionally, for 4 minutes, or until the mushrooms release their liquid. Sprinkle with the flour and cook, stirring, for 1 minute. Add the milk and cook, stirring constantly, for 3 minutes, or until thickened. Add the green beans and stir to combine.

Reduce the oven temperature to 400°F. Pour the bean mixture into the prepared baking dish. Scatter the onion rings over the top. Bake for 25 minutes, or until hot and bubbly.

Makes 8 servings

NUTRITION AT A GLANCE
Per serving: 110 calories, 3 g fat, 1 g saturated fat, 6 g protein, 15 g carbohydrate, 2 g dietary fiber, 5 mg cholesterol, 150 mg sodium

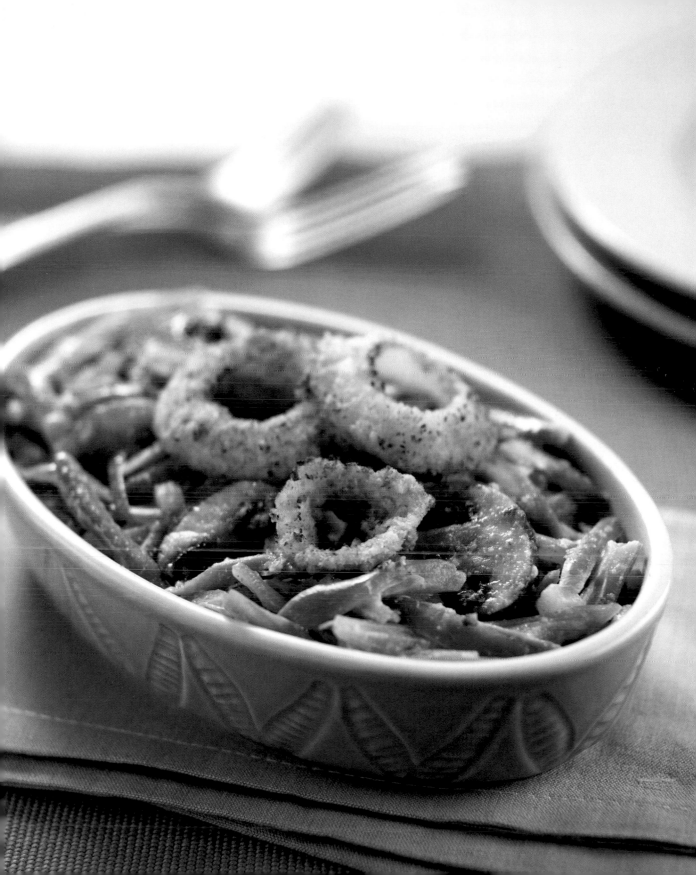

Sesame-Caraway Mixed Vegetables

Even if you think you don't care for Brussels sprouts, give them a try in this tasty recipe. The flavors of nutty sesame and anise-like caraway are a wonderful accent to these tiny bites.

- 1 tablespoon sesame seeds
- 2 teaspoons caraway seeds
- 2 teaspoons extra virgin olive oil
- 6 scallions, chopped
- 3 cups Brussels sprout halves
- 1/2 cup chicken broth
- 2 cups snow peas, trimmed
- 1 1/2 teaspoons ground black pepper
- 1/2 teaspoon low-sodium herb seasoning

Combine the sesame seeds and caraway seeds in a large nonstick skillet over medium heat. Toast the seeds, shaking the pan often, for 2 minutes, or until fragrant. Remove to a bowl.

Heat the oil in the same skillet over medium-high heat. Add the scallions and stir-fry for 1 minute. Add the Brussels sprouts and stir-fry for 2 minutes. Add the broth, cover, and simmer for 5 minutes, or until the vegetables are just tender.

Add the snow peas and cook, stirring often, for 2 minutes, or until the snow peas are crisp-tender. Stir in the seeds, pepper, and herb seasoning and cook for 1 minute.

Makes 4 servings

NUTRITION AT A GLANCE

Per serving: 90 calories, 4 g fat, 1/2 g saturated fat, 4 g protein, 11 g carbohydrate, 1/2 g dietary fiber, 0 mg cholesterol, 150 mg sodium

Sesame-Ginger Asparagus

Thin asparagus always makes an elegant side dish. Sprinkled with a hint of red-pepper flakes, the presentation is quite impressive. This dish is lovely served with a fish main course.

1 1/2	pounds thin asparagus, trimmed and cut diagonally into 2" pieces
1	tablespoon canola oil
1	tablespoon chopped fresh ginger
1	tablespoon light soy sauce
1/4	teaspoon crushed red-pepper flakes
1	teaspoon sesame oil
1	teaspoon sesame seeds

Bring 1/4" water to a boil in a large nonstick skillet over high heat. Add the asparagus and return to a boil. Reduce the heat to low, cover, and simmer for 5 minutes, or until crisp-tender. Drain and cool briefly under cold running water. Wipe the skillet dry with a paper towel.

Heat the canola oil in the same skillet over high heat. Add the asparagus, ginger, soy sauce, and red-pepper flakes and cook for 2 minutes, or until heated through. Remove from the heat and stir in the sesame oil and sesame seeds.

Makes 4 servings

NUTRITION AT A GLANCE

Per serving: 90 calories, 5 g fat, 1/2 g saturated fat, 4 g protein, 8 g carbohydrate, 4 g dietary fiber, 0 mg cholesterol, 160 mg sodium

"Fried" Green Tomatoes

You don't have to be from the South to appreciate this traditional Southern recipe, and these tomatoes aren't fried in the traditional sense of the dish. They're sautéed in a little bit of canola oil. Enjoy these as a side dish, or whip up a batch to have "just because."

- 1/2 cup whole wheat flour
- 1/2 cup finely chopped pecans
- 1 1/2 teaspoons ground black pepper
- 6 large green tomatoes, cut into 1/2" slices
- 2 tablespoons canola oil
- 1 tablespoon chopped fresh basil or 1/4 teaspoon dried

In a shallow bowl, combine the flour, pecans, and pepper. Dip the tomatoes into the mixture, turning to coat both sides.

Heat the oil in a large, heavy skillet over medium-high heat. Working in batches, add the tomatoes in a single layer. Reduce the heat to low and cook slowly until they are brown on one side. Turn the tomatoes carefully and cook until the inside is tender and the second side is brown. Remove each slice as it is finished and place on a warm serving dish. Repeat to cook all the tomatoes.

Pour the pan drippings over the tomatoes and sprinkle with the basil.

Makes 6 servings

NUTRITION AT A GLANCE

Per serving: 190 calories, 12 g fat, 1 g saturated fat, 5 g protein, 18 g carbohydrate, 4 g dietary fiber, 0 mg cholesterol, 25 mg sodium

Cheesy Baked Artichokes

Artichokes baked gratin-style are creamy and delicious. Using the frozen hearts makes this recipe a breeze to prepare.

2 packages (9 ounces each) frozen artichoke hearts

1 tablespoon lemon juice

3 tablespoons ground pecans

2 tablespoons grated Parmesan cheese

1 teaspoon dried Italian seasoning, crushed

1 clove garlic, minced

1 teaspoon extra virgin olive oil

Preheat the oven to 375°F. Coat a 9" glass pie plate with cooking spray.

Place the artichokes in a colander and rinse well with cold water to separate. Drain well, then pat dry with paper towels. Place in the prepared pie plate and sprinkle with the lemon juice.

In a small bowl, combine the pecans, cheese, Italian seasoning, garlic, and oil. Sprinkle the mixture evenly over the artichokes.

Bake for 15 minutes, or until the topping is golden.

Makes 4 servings

NUTRITION AT A GLANCE

Per serving: 110 calories, 6 g fat, 1 g saturated fat, 5 g protein, 12 g carbohydrate, 8 g dietary fiber, 0 mg cholesterol, 170 mg sodium

Nutty Summer Squash with Asiago Cheese

Summer squash couldn't be better! Chopped walnuts and Asiago, an Italian cheese with a nutty, rich flavor, add a surprise crunch to this delightful veggie dish.

2	teaspoons trans-free margarine
2	large cloves garlic, minced
1	medium zucchini, cut into 3" strips
1	medium yellow summer squash, cut into 3" spears
2	tablespoons chicken or vegetable broth
1/8	teaspoon salt
1/8	teaspoon ground black pepper
1/4	cup chopped walnuts, toasted
1/3	cup (1 1/2 ounces) shredded Asiago cheese

Melt the margarine in a large nonstick skillet over medium-low heat. Add the garlic and cook, stirring constantly, for 1 minute, or until soft.

Add the zucchini, yellow squash, broth, salt, and pepper. Bring to a simmer over medium heat. Cover and simmer, stirring occasionally, for 6 minutes, or until the zucchini and squash are tender. Remove from the heat. Sprinkle with the walnuts and cheese.

Makes 4 servings

NUTRITION AT A GLANCE

Per serving: 120 calories, 9 g fat, 2 1/2 g saturated fat, 5 g protein, 5 g carbohydrate, 2 g dietary fiber, 10 mg cholesterol, 140 mg sodium

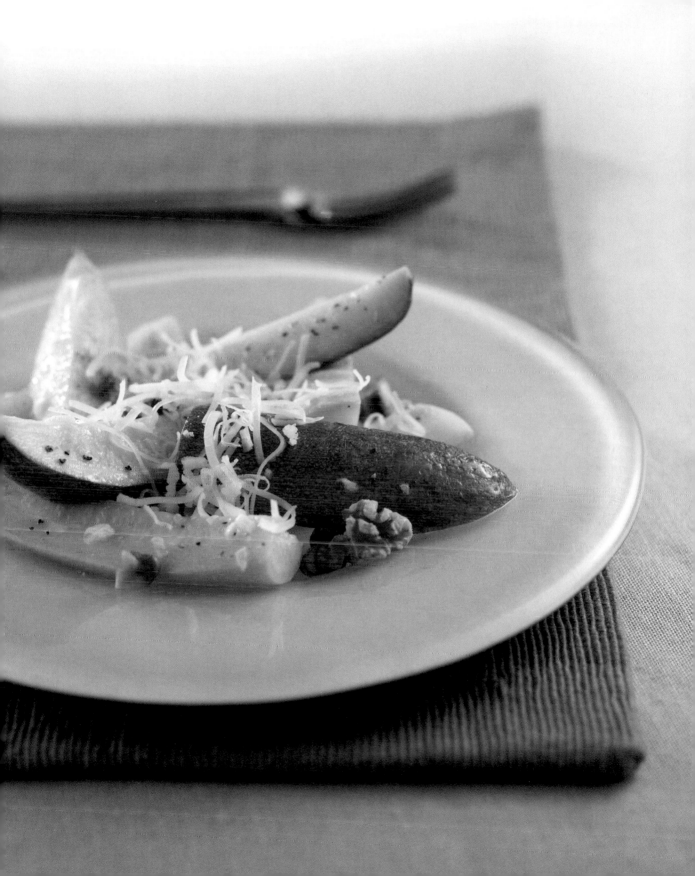

Surprise South Beach Mashed "Potatoes"

This was one of the most popular recipes in the first book, so I felt it deserved a reprise here. You won't believe how many people you'll fool with this recipe.

> 4 cups cauliflower florets
> 2 tablespoons trans-free butter spray
> 1 ounce fat-free half-and-half
>   Pinch of salt
>   Pinch of ground black pepper

Place a steamer basket in a large saucepan with 1/2 cup water. Place the cauliflower in the steamer and bring to a boil over high heat. Reduce the heat to medium, cover, and cook for 4 minutes, or until crisp-tender. Puree in a food processor, adding the butter spray and the half-and-half. Season with salt and pepper.

Makes 4 servings

NUTRITION AT A GLANCE

Per serving: 60 calories, 1 1/2 g fat, 1/2 g saturated fat, 3 g protein, 11 g carbohydrate, 3 g dietary fiber, 5 mg cholesterol, 105 mg sodium

Roasted-Pepper Cream

The heat from the peppers merges perfectly with the coolness of the sour cream.

1 jar (7 ounces) roasted red peppers, drained

2 tablespoons fat-free sour cream

1 teaspoon apple cider vinegar

Salt

Ground black pepper

In a blender or food processor, combine the peppers, sour cream, vinegar, and salt and pepper to taste. Refrigerate until ready to serve.

Makes about 1 cup

NUTRITION AT A GLANCE

Per 2 tablespoons: 5 calories, 0 g fat, 0 g saturated fat, 0 g protein, 1 g carbohydrate, 0 g dietary fiber, 0 mg cholesterol, 45 mg sodium

Eggplant "Spaghetti" Sauce

I created this sauce to serve over cooked and shredded spaghetti squash. If you have some of this sauce left after having your squash, then use the leftover sauce with any of the veggies on the acceptable list.

1 small eggplant, cut lengthwise into 1/2" slices

1 tablespoon extra virgin olive oil

1 small onion, chopped

1 clove garlic, minced

1 can (28 ounces) plum tomatoes

2 tablespoons tomato paste

2 tablespoons chopped fresh basil

Preheat the broiler.

Lightly coat the eggplant slices with olive oil cooking spray. Place on a broiler-pan rack and broil until eggplant slices are brown on both sides. Remove the eggplant slices from the oven and cut into 1" pieces.

Heat the oil in a 3-quart saucepan over medium heat. Add the onion and garlic and cook for 3 minutes, or until tender. Stir in the tomatoes (with juice), tomato paste, and basil. Cook, stirring to break up the tomatoes, for 5 minutes, or until the mixture begins to boil. Reduce the heat to low, partially cover, and simmer, stirring occasionally, for 15 minutes. Add the eggplant, stir to combine, and simmer for another 5 minutes. (Keeps covered in the refrigerator for 1 week.)

Makes 4 servings (5 cups)

NUTRITION AT A GLANCE

Per serving: 110 calories, 3 1/2 g fat, 0 g saturated fat, 4 g protein, 15 g carbohydrate, 4 g dietary fiber, 0 mg cholesterol, 370 mg sodium

JOE'S STONE CRAB

11 Washington Avenue, Miami Beach

CHEF ANDRE BIENVENU

THIS HOUSE DRESSING IS ONE OF THE MOST POPULAR
THINGS ON THE MENU AT *JOE'S STONE CRAB*.

Sweet Onion Dressing

PHASE 3

1/2	medium Vidalia onion, roasted
8	cloves garlic, chopped
1/4	cup chopped parsley
2	tablespoons sugar
1/2	cup Dijon mustard
2	cups extra virgin olive oil
1/4	cup white wine vinegar
1/2	cup water
1	teaspoon kosher salt
1	teaspoon black pepper

Preheat the grill or preheat the oven to 400°F.

Grill the onion until light brown. Place in a food processor and pulse until finely chopped. Add the garlic, parsley, sugar, and mustard and process. Slowly add the oil. Add the vinegar, water, salt, and pepper and process until well-combined.

Makes 16 (1/4 cup) servings

NUTRITION AT A GLANCE

Per 1/4 cup: 270 calories, 28 g fat, 4 g saturated fat, 1/2 g protein, 7 g carbohydrate, 0 g dietary fiber, 0 mg cholesterol, 310 mg sodium

South Beach Tomato Sauce

You can use this light tomato sauce in any recipe that calls for a red sauce or simply as a topping for chicken or fish.

1/4 cup extra virgin olive oil

1/2 onion, finely chopped

  1 can (28 ounces) peeled Italian tomatoes

1/4 cup dry white wine (optional)

  2 cloves garlic, minced

  4 leaves fresh basil, chopped

  2 tablespoons chopped parsley leaves

1/2 teaspoon sugar substitute

  Pinch of ground red pepper

1/4 cup canned, drained, pitted ripe olives, coarsely chopped

Heat the oil in a medium saucepan over medium heat. Add the onion and cook, stirring occasionally, for 3 minutes, or until soft. Add the tomatoes (with juice), wine, garlic, basil, parsley, sugar substitute, and pepper. Reduce the heat to low and simmer for 1 hour. Add the olives and simmer for 3 minutes longer. Refrigerate until serving. (Keeps covered in the refrigerator for 1 week.)

Makes about 2 cups

NUTRITION AT A GLANCE

Per 1/4 cup: 100 calories, 7 g fat, 1 g saturated fat, 1 g protein, 5 g carbohydrate, 1 g dietary fiber, 0 mg cholesterol, 220 mg sodium

South Beach Green Goddess Dressing

Here's another South Beach twist on a classic recipe from the '70s.

1/2 cup mayonnaise

1/2 cup fat-free sour cream

1 ounce chopped anchovy fillets

1/4 cup chopped parsley

3 scallions, chopped

1 tablespoon white wine vinegar

1/2 teaspoon salt

1/8 teaspoon garlic powder

1/8 teaspoon ground black pepper

In a small bowl, combine the mayonnaise, sour cream, anchovies, parsley, scallions, vinegar, salt, garlic powder, and pepper and mix well. Place in a covered container and refrigerate until ready to serve. (Keeps covered in the refrigerator for 1 week.)

Makes about 1 cup

NUTRITION AT A GLANCE

Per tablespoon: 120 calories, 12 g fat, 1 1/2 g saturated fat, 2 g protein, 3 g carbohydrate, 0 g dietary fiber, 15 mg cholesterol, 370 mg sodium

South Beach Condiments

When watching what you eat, it's easy to forget about what goes *on top* of what you eat. After all, amid the delights of a cheeseburger, fries, and soda, how dangerous do a few squirts of ketchup seem? But we ignore these toppings at our own risk, because condiments, dressings, and so on can pack their own bad carb punch. This is especially true today, when we're enticed by the endless array of sauces found in supermarkets and restaurants. We've gone way beyond the basic trio of ketchup, mustard, and mayo. Young diners who have been raised in the fast-food era would be lost without their dipping sauces—they wouldn't *think* of ordering chicken tenders, for instance, without something tasty to dunk them into. And invariably, today's most popular condiments are laden with sugar or other sweeteners. Even some savory sauces and toppings now come with a load of bad carbs.

Ketchup, by dint of its popularity, is a prime diet-buster. It isn't meant to sweeten your food, and it does taste mostly of tomato, vinegar, and spices. But examine the label: Right up there near the top of the list, you'll find high-fructose corn syrup and other forms of sugar. In a single serving of 1 tablespoon, you find 4 grams of sugar—more than in a Hershey's kiss, which contains 3 grams of sugar.

Mustard, on the other hand, is a perfectly healthy condiment. It has no carbs or fat to speak of, and it enhances the flavor of food, which is a good objective. Still, there is a way to make mustard hazardous. One of today's most popular varieties is honey mustard, which contains a substantial amount of sugar. Examine the labels and compare: Regular mustard has no sugar whatsoever; in honey mustard, you may find sugar, honey, and molasses among the ingredients. It's used most often as a dipping sauce and in salad dressings.

Mayonnaise has a bad reputation because of the cholesterol and calories from the fats and oils it contains. But today, most brands use canola or olive oil, so mayo can now be considered part of a healthy diet. It is a good source of vitamin E, plus it's filling and makes food taste good.

Barbecue sauces usually fall into two categories: savory (vinegar-based) or sweet (which contains brown sugar, molasses, or corn syrup). Guess which kind is most popular these days? Hands down, it's the sweet. And even the vinegar-based variety is now made with sweeteners. Added sugars show up unexpectedly nowadays in everything from steak sauce, which can also contain raisins for sweetness, to seafood cocktail sauce.

As we've noted, honey-based dipping sauces are all the rage these days, thanks to the fast-food influence on our eating habits. These toppings are part of what make fast-food chicken so bad for people trying to lose weight. One alternative is a no-carb, sugar-free honey vinaigrette salad dressing, which is available from several different manufacturers. It's not as rich as the high-carb stuff, but it tastes just as good.

One obvious solution to the condiment problems is simply to stick with ones without sugar or seek out brands made with sugar substitutes. But you can also make your own. For instance, you can easily make ketchup that tastes good and keeps to the South Beach Diet. For South Beach Ketchup as well as other delicious homemade condiments, see the recipes beginning on page 239.

Herbed Vinaigrette

This tasty vinaigrette is sure to spice up your salads.

- 1/2 cup white wine vinegar
- 1/2 cup extra virgin olive oil
- 2 tablespoons chopped fresh basil
- 2 tablespoons chopped fresh tarragon
- 2 tablespoons chopped parsley
- 2 tablespoons chopped fresh marjoram
- 2 teaspoons chopped fresh oregano
- 2 tablespoons drained and chopped capers
- 1 teaspoon Dijon mustard
- 1/2 teaspoon sugar substitute
- Ground black pepper (optional)

In a jar with a tightly fitting lid, combine the vinegar, oil, basil, tarragon, parsley, marjoram, oregano, capers, mustard, sugar substitute, and pepper, if using. Close the jar tightly and shake vigorously. Refrigerate until serving. (Keeps covered in the refrigerator for 1 week.)

Makes 1 1/2 cups

NUTRITION AT A GLANCE
Per tablespoon: 90 calories, 9 g fat, 1 1/2 g saturated fat, 0 g protein, 1 g carbohydrate, 0 g dietary fiber, 0 mg cholesterol, 55 mg sodium

South Beach Barbecue Sauce

- 1 can (8 ounces) tomato sauce
- 2 tablespoons white vinegar
- 1 teaspoon Worcestershire sauce
- 1 teaspoon mustard powder
- 2 teaspoons chopped parsley
- 1/4 teaspoon salt
- 1/8 teaspoon ground black pepper
- 1/8 teaspoon garlic powder

In a resealable container, combine the tomato sauce, vinegar, Worcestershire sauce, mustard powder, parsley, salt, pepper, and garlic powder. (Keeps covered in the refrigerator for 1 week.)

Makes about 1 cup

NUTRITION AT A GLANCE
Per 2 tablespoons: 21 calories, 0 g fat, 0 g saturated fat, 1/2 g protein, 6 g carbohydrate, 1/2 g dietary fiber, 0 mg cholesterol, 290 mg sodium

South Beach Cocktail Sauce

- 1 can (8 ounces) tomato sauce
- 1 tablespoon lemon juice
- 1 teaspoon Worcestershire sauce
- 1/2 teaspoon onion salt
- 1 teaspoon chopped parsley
- 1 teaspoon prepared horseradish
- 1/8 teaspoon garlic powder

In a large pot over medium heat, combine the tomato sauce, lemon juice, Worcestershire sauce, onion salt, parsley, horseradish, and garlic powder. Simmer for 5 minutes. Refrigerate until serving. (Keeps covered in the refrigerator for 1 week.)

Makes 1 cup

NUTRITION AT A GLANCE

Per 2 tablespoons: 10 calories, 0 g fat, 0 g saturated fat, 0 g protein, 3 g carbohydrate, 0 g dietary fiber, 0 mg cholesterol, 310 mg sodium

South Beach Teriyaki Sauce

1/2 cup light soy sauce

1/2 cup dry sherry

1/4 cup sugar-free pancake syrup

1/4 cup ground arrowroot

3 tablespoons red wine vinegar

4 cloves garlic, crushed

1 teaspoon ground ginger

1/4 teaspoon hot-pepper sauce

In a food processor, combine the soy sauce, sherry, syrup, arrowroot, vinegar, garlic, ginger, and hot-pepper sauce. Pulse until smooth. (Keeps covered in the refrigerator for 1 week.)

Makes 1 1/2 cups

NUTRITION AT A GLANCE

Per 2 tablespoons: 30 calories, 0 g fat, 0 g saturated fat, 1 g protein, 5 g carbohydrate, 0 g dietary fiber, 0 mg cholesterol, 420 mg sodium

South Beach Ketchup

  1 can (8 ounces) tomato sauce
3/4 cup tomato paste
  2 tablespoons sugar substitute
  2 teaspoons onion powder
  2 teaspoons light soy sauce
1/2 teaspoon ground cloves
1/2 teaspoon ground allspice
1 1/2 tablespoons malt vinegar

In a large pot over medium heat, combine the tomato sauce, tomato paste, sugar substitute, onion powder, soy sauce, cloves, allspice, and vinegar. Simmer for 5 minutes. Refrigerate until serving. (Keeps covered in the refrigerator for 1 week.)

Makes about 1 cup

NUTRITION AT A GLANCE

Per 2 tablespoons: 45 calories, 0 g fat, 0 g saturated fat, 2 g protein, 10 g carbohydrate, 2 g dietary fiber, 0 mg cholesterol, 390 mg sodium

South Beach Ballpark Mustard

This recipe requires a little bit of effort, but homemade mustard, like so many things, really does taste better than store-bought.

3/4 cup water

1/4 cup mustard seeds

1/4 cup + 2 tablespoons mustard powder

1/4 teaspoon dried tarragon

1 tablespoon ground turmeric

1/2 cup tarragon vinegar

1/2 cup dry white wine

1 tablespoon canola oil

1/4 cup sugar substitute

2 cloves garlic, minced

1/4 teaspoon ground allspice

1/4 teaspoon ground cinnamon

1/4 teaspoon ground cloves

1/2 teaspoon arrowroot

In a small bowl, combine water, mustard seeds, mustard powder, tarragon, and turmeric.

In a medium saucepan combine the vinegar, wine, oil, sugar substitute, garlic, allspice, cinnamon, and cloves. Bring to a boil over medium–high heat and simmer for 5 minutes.

In a blender or food processor, combine the mustard and vinegar mixtures and blend for 2 minutes. Return the mixture to the saucepan and heat on low heat for 5 minutes. Stir in the arrowroot to thicken. (Keeps covered in the refrigerator for 1 week.)

Makes about 1 1/2 cups

NUTRITION AT A GLANCE

Per tablespoon: 35 calories, 2 g fat, 0 g saturated fat, 1 g protein, 3 g carbohydrate, 0 g dietary fiber, 0 mg cholesterol, 0 mg sodium

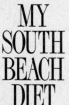

I'M LIVING PROOF OF THE CONNECTION BETWEEN DIABETES, WEIGHT LOSS, AND HEART HEALTH.

I have tried every diet out there, both fad and physician-prescribed, and I've always had the same disappointing outcome. Because previous diets did not fit into my normal, everyday life, I would struggle and give up quickly. At age 57, I weighed 279 pounds and was taking medications and daily insulin shots to control the type 2 diabetes I have had for 10 years. Since starting the South Beach Diet, my health has rapidly improved. A 25-pound weight loss!—and feeling more in control of my life is just an added bonus.

Before South Beach, I started Weight Watchers with my daughter and did pretty well, losing 8 pounds in 8 or

9 weeks, but then I gained 5 pounds back in the following 2 weeks. Talk about disappointment! At this point, I started to believe that I was the typical "hopelessly overweight" person, who would never lose any more than 10 pounds.

That's when I checked the Prevention.com Message Forum and became inspired by what people were saying about the South Beach Diet. Just 4 days after jumping onto the "Beach," I weighed in and found that I had dropped 7.8 pounds. I was ecstatic! Three days after that, I had an appointment with my nurse practitioner and I had lost another 1.5 pounds! She then took me off two of my medications and told me that if my blood sugar stayed within normal limits, I could wean myself off the insulin. I floated out of her office that day.

Since starting the diet, I have stayed on Phase 1, adding back fruit but not pasta, bread, or rice. It's good to know that I could have some if I wanted, but I like the way I feel without them.

Although I've had a couple of minor setbacks, I plan on continuing just what I'm doing until I get to 175 pounds. It really doesn't look that far away or hopeless to me any more.

I still go to the WW meetings for the personal support and accountability, and I also participate in the South Beach discussion forum online. I think emotional support is really essential in any success. We are all educating ourselves about a new way to live, and any words of wisdom are invaluable.

Overall, the actual pounds lost, while significant, are but a tiny measure of the health changes I've actually experienced. I'm living proof of the connection between diabetes and weight. —*CHERYL O.*

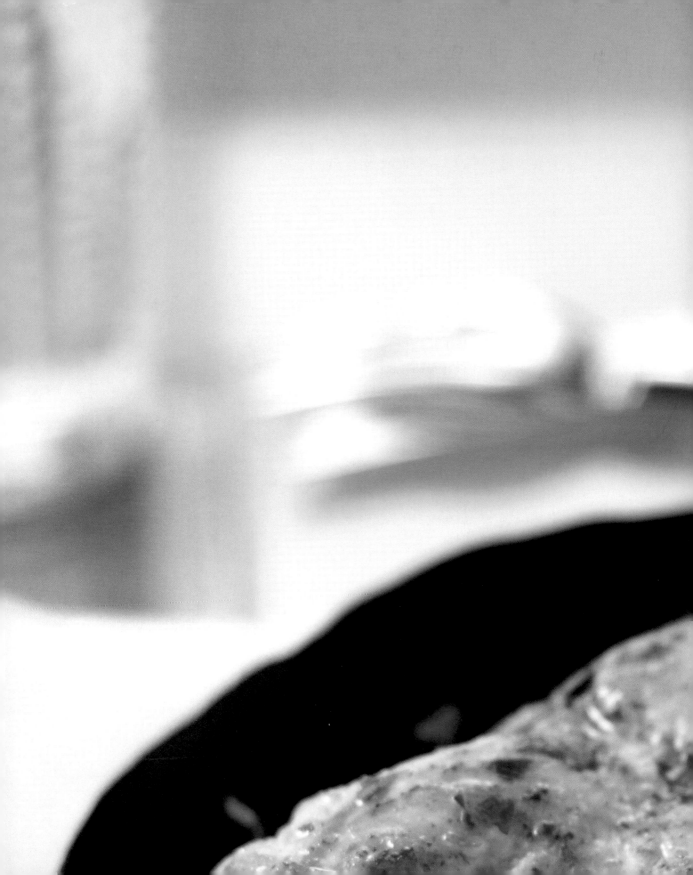

FISH, SHELLFISH, AND POULTRY

Eating fish has practically become a form of self-medication, thanks to all the news stories about the health benefits of salmon, tuna, and the rest. It's absolutely true that three or four meals a week of these so-called oily fish (mackerel or sardines, too) can help prevent heart attacks. The omega-3 fatty acids these fish contain keep blood platelets from forming sticky clumps that block arteries.

Similarly, we've all become faithful fans of skinless white-meat chicken and turkey for reasons of weight control and cardiovascular health. But making these wise dietary moves doesn't require us to sacrifice anything when it comes to eating well.

The South Beach Diet reflects its Florida origins especially in its fish and seafood recipes. There's a terrific recipe for ceviche and one for perch "breaded" with crushed smoked almonds that can be adapted to any kind of fish fillet.

247

Zesty Crab Cakes with Creamy Pepper Sauce

Though you can use canned crabmeat if it's in your cupboard, fresh lump crabmeat is far superior in these crab cakes. Drizzled with a creamy roasted pepper sauce, this is one recipe you'll make again and again.

Creamy Pepper Sauce

- 2 whole jarred roasted red peppers, drained
- 1/2 cup mayonnaise
  Ground black pepper

Crab Cakes

- 1 teaspoon extra virgin olive oil
- 1/2 onion, finely chopped
- 1 rib celery, finely chopped
- 1 egg white
- 2 tablespoons ground walnuts
- 2 tablespoons chopped Italian parsley
- 2 tablespoons mayonnaise
- 1 tablespoon lemon juice
- 1 1/2 teaspoons crab boil seasoning, such as Old Bay
- 2 teaspoons Worcestershire sauce
- 1/2 teaspoon mustard powder
- 1/4 teaspoon celery seeds, crushed
- 1/2 teaspoon ground paprika
- 1 pound lump crabmeat, flaked and drained

1/2 teaspoon hot-pepper sauce

1 cup fresh whole wheat bread crumbs

Sprig Italian parsley, for garnish

To make the sauce: Puree the roasted peppers in a food processor or blender. Add the mayonnaise and black pepper as desired and process briefly to combine. Transfer to a small bowl.

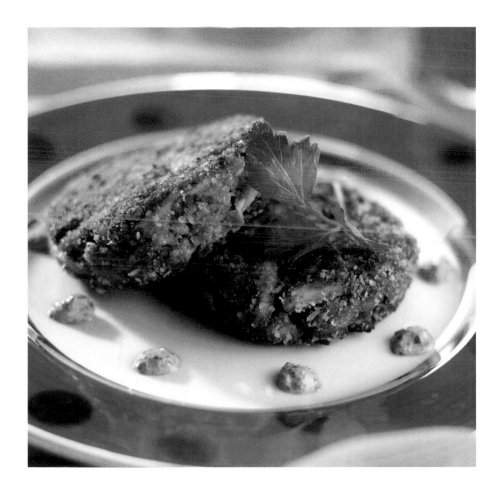

To make the crab cakes: Heat the oil in a medium nonstick skillet over medium-high heat. Add the onion and celery and cook for 5 minutes, or until soft. Remove to a large bowl.

Stir in the egg white, walnuts, parsley, mayonnaise, lemon juice, crab boil seasoning, Worcestershire sauce, mustard powder, celery seeds, and paprika. Blend with a fork. Stir in the crabmeat and hot-pepper sauce. Mix thoroughly. Form into 8 patties. Place the bread crumbs in a shallow bowl. Roll the patties in the bread crumbs to coat completely.

Heat a large nonstick skillet coated with cooking spray over medium-high heat. Working in batches if necessary, add the crab cakes and cook for 2 minutes. Cover and cook for 1 minute longer, or until browned on the bottom. Coat the tops with cooking spray and turn over. Cook for 2 minutes longer, uncovered, or until golden brown. Serve with the sauce dolloped in dots on the plate. Garnish with the parsley.

Makes 4 servings

NUTRITION AT A GLANCE

Per serving: 470 calories, 34 g fat, 5 g saturated fat, 24 g protein, 17 g carbohydrate, 2 g dietary fiber, 115 mg cholesterol, 800 mg sodium

Ceviche

Ceviche, seviche, and cebiche are all names for the Peruvian/Ecuadorian method of cooking fish in the acid of a fruit. Many believe that this delightfully light and simple cooking method was first devised by the Incas.

- 1 pound mahi mahi or any white, firm-fleshed, fresh fish, washed and cut into small cubes
- 1/2 cup fresh lime juice
- 1 clove garlic, crushed
- 1/4–1/2 teaspoon hot-pepper sauce
-   Salt
-   Coarsely ground black pepper
- 1 large onion, finely chopped
- 1 red bell pepper, cut into strips
- 1 rib celery, finely chopped
- 1/2 cup chopped fresh cilantro

Place the fish in a large glass bowl. Add the lime juice, garlic, and hot-pepper sauce, and sprinkle with salt and black pepper. Cover and refrigerate for 1 hour. Add the onion, bell pepper, celery, and cilantro. Cover and refrigerate for 1 hour longer.

Serve chilled in martini glasses for an elegant look.

Makes 4 servings

NUTRITION AT A GLANCE

Per serving: 131 calories, 1 g fat, 0 g saturated fat, 22 g protein, 9 g carbohydrate, 2 g dietary fiber, 83 mg cholesterol, 123 mg sodium

From the Menu of . . .

THE LOEWS
MIAMI BEACH HOTEL

1601 Collins Avenue, Miami Beach

EXECUTIVE CHEF MARC EHRLER

The Loews Miami Beach Hotel was the first
to open on the hotel strip on Collins Avenue.
It helped lay the groundwork for
the Miami Beach renaissance.

Grilled Mahi Mahi on Chopped Salad
with Olive Oil Lemon Vinaigrette

PHASE 1

1	mahi mahi fillet (7 ounces)
	Extra virgin olive oil
	Salt
	Pepper
1	cup iceberg lettuce, torn
1	cup arugula leaves
1	small cucumber, sliced
1/2	cup jarred marinated artichokes
1/4	cup chopped red bell pepper
2	teaspoons finely chopped yellow bell pepper

1/4 cup red onion, thinly sliced

1 tablespoon fresh basil, roughly chopped

1 tablespoon extra virgin olive oil

2 tablespoons fresh lemon juice

Salt

Black pepper

Preheat the grill.

Place the mahi mahi on a small plate. Drizzle the mahi mahi with olive oil and season with salt and pepper. Place the mahi mahi at 10 o'clock for 2 1/2 minutes. Turn the mahi mahi to 2 o'clock. Cook for another 2 1/2 minutes and flip over. Repeat the cooking instruction on the other side of the fish and cook until done.

In a medium mixing bowl, combine the lettuce, arugula, cucumber, artichokes, red pepper, yellow pepper, onion, and basil. Toss with the olive oil and lemon juice. Season with salt and pepper to taste. Place the salad in a serving dish and arrange the cooked mahi mahi on top.

Makes 1 serving

NUTRITION AT A GLANCE

Per serving: 386 calories, 15 g fat, 2 g saturated fat, 42 g protein, 21 g carbohydrate, 8 g dietary fiber, 145 mg cholesterol, 231 mg sodium

Crab Royale

While dining on this rich, succulent crab, turn down the lights and light the candles, and you can feel as though you're eating at a café on the rue Royale in Paris.

2 cups (8 ounces) cooked crabmeat, drained and flaked

1 cup (4 ounces) reduced-fat shredded Cheddar cheese

1/4 cup whole wheat bread crumbs

1/4 cup mayonnaise

1/4 cup 1% milk

1 rib celery, chopped

2 tablespoons chopped pimiento

2 tablespoons chopped green bell pepper

1 teaspoon instant minced onion

1 teaspoon lemon juice

Pinch of black pepper

Pinch of salt

Preheat the oven to 350°F.

In a large bowl, combine the crabmeat, cheese, bread crumbs, mayonnaise, milk, celery, pimiento, bell pepper, onion, lemon juice, black pepper, and salt. Mix thoroughly. Spoon the mixture into 2 small baking dishes.

Bake for 15 minutes, or until lightly browned and heated through.

Makes 4 servings

NUTRITION AT A GLANCE

Per serving: 322 calories, 22 g fat, 8 g saturated fat, 22 g protein, 8 g carbohydrate, 1 g dietary fiber, 96 mg cholesterol, 546 mg sodium

MACALUSO'S
1747 Alton Road, Miami Beach

CHEF MICHAEL D'ANDREA

Macaluso's is the only Miami restaurant that serves home-cooked Italian food Staten-Island style. The menu is based on three generations of chef D'Andrea's family recipes, and everything is made from scratch

Broiled Sea Bass Staten Island Style
PHASE 1

3	tablespoons extra virgin olive oil
4	cloves garlic
10–12	ounces Chilean farm-raised sea bass, cleaned
1/4	teaspoon salt
1/4	teaspoon pepper
1/2	teaspoon paprika
1/4	teaspoon crushed red pepper
1	teaspoon fresh chopped Italian parsley
1/2	teaspoon fresh basil
1/2	lemon

Preheat the oven to 500°F.

In a blender combine the oil and garlic until well-blended.

Place the fish in a medium bowl. Pour the oil mixture over the fish. Marinate well, for about 30 minutes.

Remove the fish from the bowl and place in a small broiling tray, about 1" larger than the fish. Sprinkle the fish with the salt, pepper, paprika, and red pepper.

In a small bowl combine the parsley and basil. Sprinkle over the fish. Squeeze the lemon juice over the fish.

Bake the fish for 25 to 30 minutes.

Makes 2 servings

NUTRITION AT A GLANCE

Per serving: 340 calories, 24 g fat, 3 1/2 g saturated fat, 27 g protein, 4 g carbohydrate, 0 g dietary fiber, 60 mg cholesterol, 390 mg sodium

Five-Spice Salmon

Sometimes in life we want to experience everything rolled into one. In the creation of five-spice powder, the Chinese gave us that chance. With fennel, cloves, cinnamon, star anise, and Szechuan peppercorns, we get to taste sour, bitter, sweet, pungent, and salty all at once. If you've never tried five-spice powder before, you might want to halve the amount, or your taste buds might just blow a fuse!

1 1/2	teaspoons finely grated lime peel
3	tablespoons fresh lime juice
2	teaspoons extra virgin olive oil
4	teaspoons finely chopped fresh ginger
1	teaspoon Chinese five-spice powder
1/2	teaspoon sugar substitute
1	pound salmon steaks, cut into 4 equal-size pieces
8	cups fresh baby spinach leaves
2	cloves garlic, pressed

In a 2-quart dish, combine the lime peel, lime juice, 1 teaspoon of the oil, the ginger, five-spice powder, and sugar substitute. Add the salmon and turn to coat. Cover and refrigerate for 30 minutes.

In a 3-quart microwaveable dish, combine the spinach, garlic, and the remaining 1 teaspoon oil, tossing gently. Cover with plastic wrap and microwave for 2 minutes, or until the spinach has wilted. Drain and keep warm.

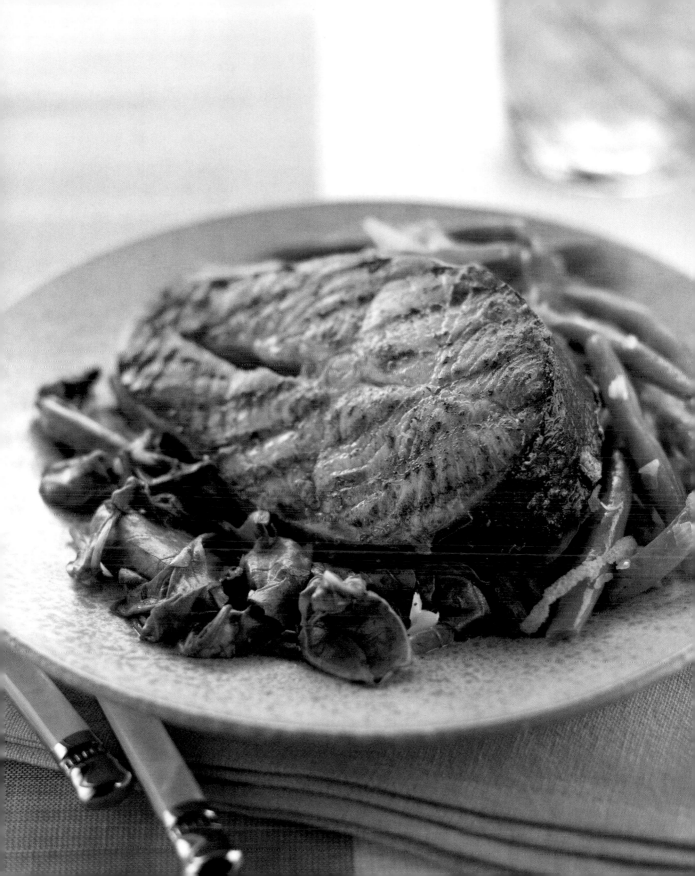

Lightly oil a grill rack. Preheat the grill to medium-high.

Remove the salmon from the marinade and place on the grill rack. Brush the salmon with additional marinade. Close the grill cover and cook for 4 minutes. Open the grill cover, turn the salmon, and brush with marinade. Close the cover and cook for 4 minutes longer, or until the salmon flakes easily. Discard any remaining marinade.

To serve, evenly divide the spinach among 4 serving plates and center the salmon on the spinach beds.

Makes 4 servings

NUTRITION AT A GLANCE

Per serving: 251 calories, 15 g fat, 3 g saturated fat, 24 g protein, 5 g carbohydrate, 2 g dietary fiber, 67 mg cholesterol, 213 mg sodium

Broiled Salmon with Creamy Lemon Sauce

This deceptively simple salmon entrée includes a sinfully rich-tasting lemony sauce that will impress every time. For best results, squeeze your own fresh lemon juice.

1	tablespoon extra virgin olive oil
1	clove garlic, minced
1/4	cup lemon juice
2	tablespoons capers
1	teaspoon lemon-pepper seasoning
1/2	cup fat-free sour cream
1 1/2	pounds salmon fillet

Preheat the oven to 350°F. Coat a baking sheet with cooking spray.

Heat the oil in a small saucepan over medium heat. Add the garlic and cook for 1 minute. Reduce heat to low. Stir in the lemon juice, capers, and lemon-pepper seasoning and cook for 5 minutes. Add the sour cream and cook for 5 minutes, or until heated through.

Meanwhile, place the salmon on the prepared baking sheet. Bake for 20 minutes, or until the fish is just opaque. Serve with the sauce.

Makes 4 servings

NUTRITION AT A GLANCE
Per serving: 368 calories, 22 g fat, 4 g saturated fat, 35 g protein, 5 g carbohydrate, 0 g dietary fiber, 100 mg cholesterol, 383 mg sodium

Pan-Seared Pecan Grouper

Whole grain cereal flakes contribute to the coating of these marinated fillets. Pan-searing and a small amount of toasted pecans gives this very lean fish wonderful flavor.

- 3 scallions, chopped
- 3 tablespoons South Beach Teriyaki Sauce (see page 241)
- 1 large clove garlic, minced
- 1 teaspoon finely chopped fresh ginger
- 4 grouper fillets (4 ounces each)
- 3/4 cup finely ground pecans
- 1/2 cup whole grain cereal flakes, coarsely crushed
- 1/4 cup pecans, toasted and chopped
- 1 teaspoon ground black pepper
- 2 tablespoons chopped fresh basil

In a 9" × 9" glass baking dish, combine the scallions, teriyaki sauce, garlic, and ginger. Place the grouper in the marinade and turn to coat both sides. Cover and refrigerate for 1 to 2 hours.

In a pie plate, combine the ground pecans, cereal flakes, toasted pecans, and pepper. Remove the grouper from the marinade. Discard the marinade. Press each fillet into the mixture to coat all sides.

Heat a large nonstick skillet coated with cooking spray over medium-high heat. Add the grouper and cook for 3 minutes, or until golden brown on the bottom. Mist the top of the fillets with cooking spray, then turn and cook for 3 minutes more, or until the grouper flakes easily. Sprinkle with the basil.

Makes 4 servings

NUTRITION AT A GLANCE

Per serving: 319 calories, 26 g fat, 2 g saturated fat, 26 g protein, 12 g carbohydrate, 4 g dietary fiber, 42 mg cholesterol, 621 mg sodium

CHINA GRILL

404 Washington Avenue, Miami Beach

CHEF KEYVAN BEHNAM

China Grill has been a Miami hot spot since it opened in 1995. It offers funky "World fusion" cuisine and first-rate people watching.

Barbecue Salmon

PHASE 3

Salmon

- 1 1/2 pounds skin-on salmon fillet (four 6-ounce fillets)
- 3/4 cup prepared barbecue sauce
- 2 tablespoons rice wine vinegar
- 2 tablespoons finely chopped scallions
- 1 teaspoon finely chopped ginger
- Chives, chopped, for garnish

Vegetables

- 1/2 head napa cabbage
- 1/2 head radicchio
- 1 1/2 teaspoons extra virgin olive oil

1	pound oyster mushrooms, chopped
1/2	cup sake or white wine
1/4	teaspoon salt
1/4	teaspoon pepper

Chinese Mustard Sauce

2	tablespoons mayonnaise
	Dash of mustard powder
1/8	teaspoon Dijon mustard
3/4	teaspoon rice wine vinegar
1 1/2	teaspoons finely chopped scallion
	Salt
	Pepper

To make the salmon: Preheat the grill.

Leave the skin on the salmon if desired.

Place the barbecue sauce, vinegar, scallions, and ginger in a blender and mix.

Start grilling the salmon to the desired doneness and baste with barbecue sauce

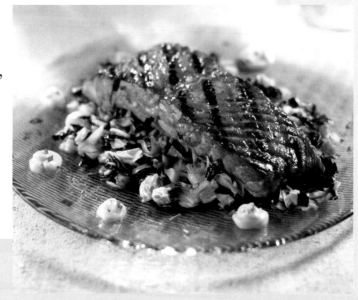

mixture as grilling. (If you like the skin, first grill skin side down until the skin is crispy, then turn over and continue basting with barbecue sauce mixture.)

To make the vegetables: Take out the hard bottom center of the greens. Slice the greens thinly. Heat a sauté pan over high heat. Add the oil and sauté the cabbage, radicchio, and mushrooms quickly. (They should stay crisp.) Before taking the vegetables out of the pan, deglaze with the sake or white wine. Add the salt and pepper.

To make the Chinese Mustard Sauce: Place the mayonnaise, mustard powder, mustard, vinegar, scallion, and salt and pepper to taste in a blender and mix.

To plate: Place sautéed vegetables in center of each plate. Put five dots of Chinese Mustard Sauce around the vegetables. Place the salmon on top of the vegetables. Sprinkle the plates with chopped chives.

Makes 4 servings

NUTRITION AT A GLANCE

Per serving: 510 calories, 27 g fat, 4 g saturated fat, 41 g protein, 19 g carbohydrate, 4 g dietary fiber, 105 mg cholesterol, 720 mg sodium

Poached Hapu'upu'u (Hawaiian Sea Bass)

If you can't get the mouthwatering meaty Hawaiian type of sea bass, replace it with whichever meaty type sea bass is available where you are. You can ask your fishmonger to save you some fish stock, or make a cup of your own with a cube of fish bouillon. Since you only need 1/4 cup, you can save the remaining 3/4 cup for another dish. Or, simply replace the stock with the same amount of water.

1	Hapu'upu'u or any meaty sea bass (8 ounces)
1/4	cup dry white wine
1/4	cup fish stock or water
1	bay leaf
1/2	clove garlic, minced
2	plum tomatoes, halved
2	scallions, chopped
1	sprig fresh thyme
	Pinch of saffron threads

Place the bass in the center of a large nonstick skillet. Cover with the wine and fish stock and place over medium heat until the liquid begins to shimmer (heat emanates from the liquid). Add the bay leaf, garlic, tomatoes, scallions, thyme, and saffron. Cover and poach for 10 minutes.

Remove the bass to a serving plate and cover with poaching liquid. Surround with the tomatoes and scallions. Remove and discard the bay leaf before serving.

Makes 2 servings

NUTRITION AT A GLANCE

Per serving: 164 calories, 22 g fat, 0 g saturated fat, 22 g protein, 6 g carbohydrate, 2 g dietary fiber, 48 mg cholesterol, 150 mg sodium

Bombay-Style Sole

Bombay-style cooking is noted for its creamy sauces and the pungent fragrance of its spices. You can also use this marinade for boneless, skinless chicken breasts—just increase the cooking time to 20 minutes.

1 cup fat-free plain yogurt
1 teaspoon curry powder
1 teaspoon ground cardamom
1 teaspoon ground paprika
1 teaspoon dried cilantro
1 1/2 pounds fillet of sole, skinned
Salt
Ground black pepper

In a blender or food processor, combine the yogurt, curry powder, cardamom, paprika, and cilantro. Process to blend.

Place the sole in a rectangular baking dish. Cover with the yogurt mixture. Cover and refrigerate for 2 to 3 hours, turning the fillets about every 30 minutes.

Preheat the oven to 350°F. Cook the sole for 10 minutes, or until it flakes easily. Season with the salt and pepper to taste.

Makes 4 servings

NUTRITION AT A GLANCE
Per serving: 160 calories, 2 g fat, 0 g saturated fat, 29 g protein, 6 g carbohydrate, 1 g dietary fiber, 70 mg cholesterol, 300 mg sodium

Florida Red Snapper

Red snapper is one of South Florida's popular fish. The only way you could enjoy this dish more would be if you caught the fish yourself.

- 2 pounds red snapper or any sea bass, cleaned
- 3 tablespoon extra virgin olive oil
- 1/8 teaspoon salt
- 1/8 teaspoon ground black pepper
- 1/4 onion, finely chopped
- 1/4 cup finely chopped celery
- 2 tablespoons finely chopped green bell pepper
- 1 scallion, chopped
- 1/2 cup pine nuts, toasted
- 2 tablespoons finely chopped parsley
- 2 tablespoons coarsely chopped almonds, toasted
- 3 thin tomato slices
- 3 thin onion slices
- 3 thin lime slices
- Salt
- Pepper
- Juice of 1/4 lime

Preheat the oven to 350°F.

Rub the fish lightly with 1 tablespoon of the oil and sprinkle the inside and outside with the salt and black pepper.

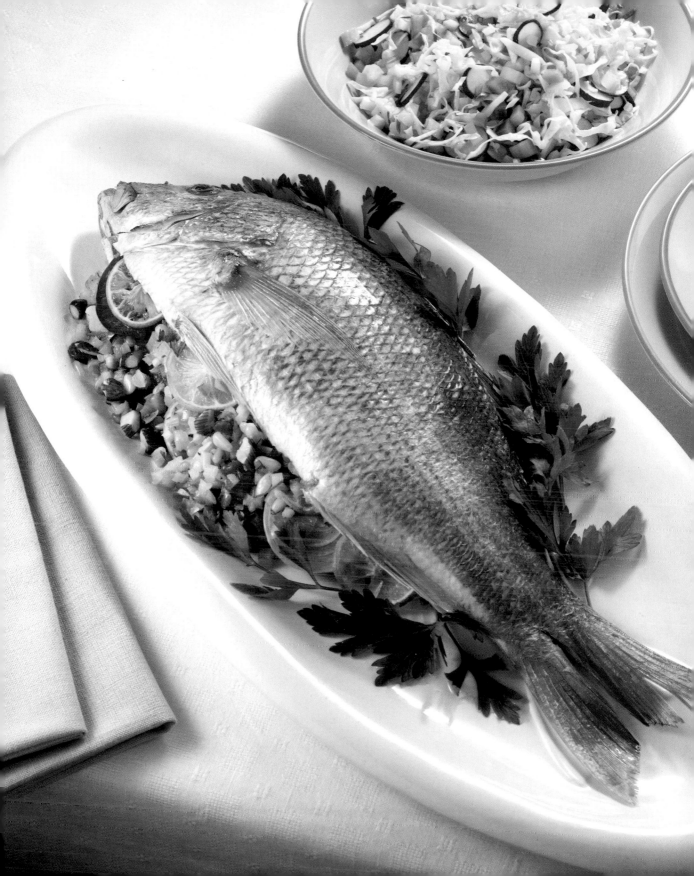

Heat the remaining 2 tablespoons oil in a small saucepan. Add the chopped onion, celery, bell pepper, and scallion and cook, stirring occasionally, for 3 minutes, or until the onion is wilted. Stir in the pine nuts, parsley, and almonds. Stuff the fish with the mixture and tie with kitchen string. Place the fish on a piece of foil and cover with alternating overlapping slices of tomato, onion, and lime. Sprinkle with salt and black pepper and drizzle with the lime juice. Bring up the edges of the foil and seal.

Bake for 30 minutes, or until the fish flakes easily. Serve with Overnight Slaw (see page 209).

Makes 4 servings

NUTRITION AT A GLANCE

Per serving: 402 calories, 19 g fat, 3 g saturated fat, 50 g protein, 6 g carbohydrate, 2 g dietary fiber, 84 mg cholesterol, 162 mg sodium

Red Snapper with Avocado Salsa

Low-fat fish with the right fats from the avocado sends this dish right up the South Beach dieter's alley. See the Vegetarian Chili with Avocado Salsa recipe on page 436 for the ingredients and preparation of the Avocado Salsa.

2 cups water

1 medium onion, sliced and separated into rings

1/4 lime, sliced

1 clove garlic, crushed

2 tablespoons chopped parsley

4 black peppercorns, crushed

1/2 teaspoon dried thyme, crushed

1/2 teaspoon dried oregano, crushed

1 whole red snapper, cleaned (about 2 pounds)

1 teaspoon salt

1 lemon, quartered

1 lime, quartered

Sprigs parsley, for garnish

In a fish poacher or a large pan, combine the water, onion, sliced lime, garlic, parsley, peppercorns, thyme, and oregano. Bring to a boil over medium-high heat, then reduce heat to low, cover, and simmer for 5 minutes.

Lightly sprinkle the fish cavity with the salt. Place the fish on cheesecloth, folding the cloth over the fish. Place on the rack in the poaching pan and immerse in the boiling poaching liquid. If there is insufficient liquid to cover the fish, bring extra water to a boil and pour over the fish until nearly covered. Cover and poach the fish for 30 minutes, or until the fish flakes easily. Remove the fish to a serving platter and cover with foil. Refrigerate until cool.

To serve, cut the fish crosswise and remove the bones. Arrange the lemon and lime quarters around the fish and spoon Avocado Salsa onto the fish. Serve with additional salsa as desired. Garnish with the parsley.

Makes 4 servings

NUTRITION AT A GLANCE
Per serving: 254 calories, 3 g fat, 1 g saturated fat, 47 g protein, 7 g carbohydrate, 2 g dietary fiber, 84 mg cholesterol, 153 mg sodium

Citrus Tuna with Fruit Skewers

Kebabs are always a hit at any backyard barbecue. Here, tangy citrus fruits are combined with juicy cherry tomatoes on skewers to accompany succulent marinated tuna. What a great reason to fire up the grill!

- 1 can (8 ounces) pineapple chunks in juice
- 2 tablespoons light soy sauce
- 1 teaspoon sesame oil
- 2 teaspoons finely chopped fresh ginger
- 1/4 teaspoon crushed red-pepper flakes
- 1 clove garlic, minced
- 1 pound tuna steaks, 3/4" to 1" thick
- 1 navel orange, peeled and cut into 8 pieces
- 4 cherry tomatoes

Drain the juice from the pineapple into a measuring cup and set the chunks aside. Add enough water to the pineapple juice to make 3/4 cup. Add the soy sauce, oil, ginger, red-pepper flakes, and garlic. Stir to combine. Set aside 2 tablespoons of marinade. Pour the remaining mixture into a zip-top plastic bag. Add the tuna and seal the bag. Shake well to coat the fish. Refrigerate for at least 30 minutes.

While tuna marinates, place the pineapple chunks, orange pieces, and tomatoes on skewers.

Coat a grill rack with cooking spray. Preheat the grill to medium.

Place the fish on the prepared grill rack and grill, brushing with the reserved marinade, for 5 minutes on each side, or until the fish flakes easily.

During the last 3 minutes of cooking, place the skewers on the grill. Grill, turning and brushing with reserved marinade, for 3 minutes, or until hot.

Makes 4 servings

NUTRITION AT A GLANCE

Per serving: 187 calories, 2 g fat, 1 g saturated fat, 26 g protein, 15 g carbohydrate, 2 g dietary fiber, 53 mg cholesterol, 347 mg sodium

Grilled Tuna with Teriyaki Glaze

This tuna will make your mouth water. Grilled to absolute perfection and brushed with a sassy teriyaki-like glaze, this is a recipe that satisfies the whole family.

- 1/4 cup light soy sauce
- 3 tablespoons dry sherry or chicken broth
- 1 tablespoon grated fresh ginger
- 3 cloves garlic, minced
- 4 tuna steaks (5 ounces each)
- 1 large mango, peeled and cut into spears
- 1 red bell pepper, quartered lengthwise

In a small bowl, combine the soy sauce, sherry or broth, ginger, and garlic. Divide the marinade into 2 medium, shallow bowls. Place the tuna in one bowl and the mango and bell pepper in the other. Turn the tuna, mango, and bell pepper to coat both sides. Cover and refrigerate for 15 minutes.

Coat a grill rack or broiler pan rack with cooking spray. Preheat the grill or broiler to medium.

Place the tuna, mango, and bell pepper on the prepared rack or pan. Discard the marinade from the tuna bowl. Grill or broil, basting occasionally with the marinade from the mango bowl, for 4 minutes per side, or until the tuna is just opaque and the

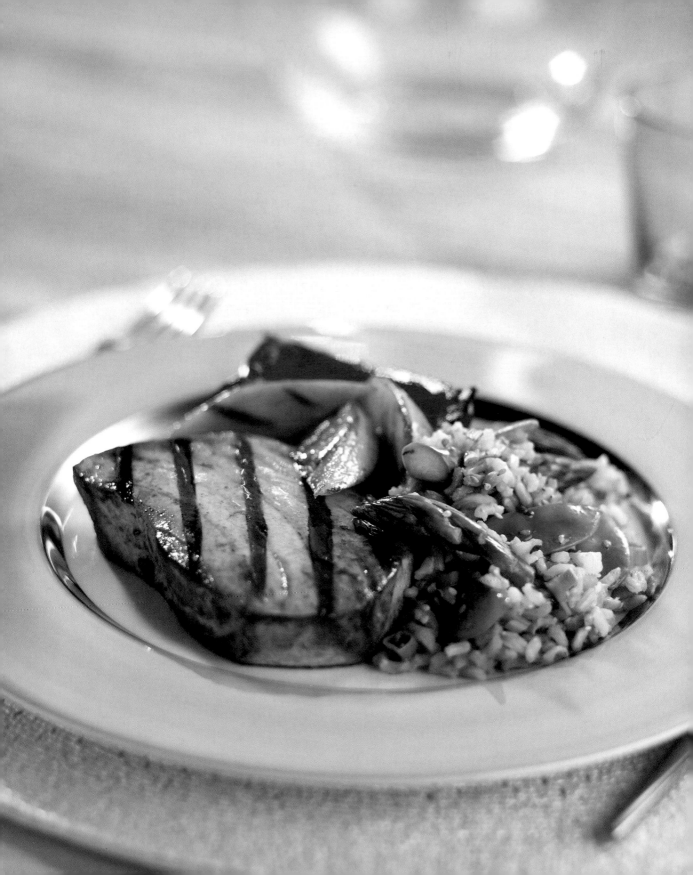

mango and bell pepper are heated through and glazed.

Makes 4 servings

NUTRITION AT A GLANCE

Per serving: 207 calories, 2 g fat, 1 g saturated fat, 33 g protein, 12 g carbohydrate, 2 g dietary fiber, 67 mg cholesterol, 509 mg sodium

From the Menu of . . .
BARTON G
THE RESTAURANT
1427 West Avenue, Miami Beach

CHEF TED MENDEZ

COMBINING "FINE" DINING WITH "FUN" DINING, *BARTON G THE RESTAURANT* MAKES EACH MEAL AN EXPERIENCE. IN MAY 2003, CONDÉ NAST TRAVELER NAMED *BARTON G THE RESTAURANT* ONE OF THE "75 TOP NEW RESTAURANTS FROM BOSTON TO BEIJING."

Shellfish in a Pot
PHASE 3

1	sprig thyme, chopped
1	bay leaf
1	cup chopped carrot
1	cup chopped celery
1	cup chopped onion
1/2	cup sliced shallots
3	artichoke bottoms with stems
2	tablespoons extra virgin olive oil

3	tablespoons trans-free margarine or butter
1 1/2	cups mixed green and wax beans, cut diagonally and blanched
2	warm-water lobster tails, split (6 ounces each)
12	fresh prawns or langostinos
4	extra-large shrimp
1/2	cup chopped basil
5	baby zucchini, sliced
1	cup leek, julienned
1	cup fennel, julienned
1	tablespoon pickling spice
16	ounces shrimp stock (from boiled shellfish shells)
4	sprigs basil
	Juice of 1 lemon

In a saucepan over low heat, caramelize the thyme, bay leaf, carrot, celery, onion, shallots, and artichokes in the oil. Add 1 tablespoon margarine or butter and continue to cook over low heat for 25 to 35 minutes or until the artichokes are tender. Remove the artichokes, strain the cooking fluid, and reserve. Cut the artichokes into small wedges.

Reheat the cooking liquid in a decorative iron or clay pot. Add the beans and heat for 2 minutes.

Whisk in the remaining 2 tablespoons margarine or butter and add the lobster, prawns or langostinos, shrimp, and chopped basil. Cover tightly and simmer for 6 to 8 minutes. Remove from the heat and keep covered for 4 additional minutes.

Place the zucchini, leek, and fennel in a steamer basket. Add the pickling spice. Poach the vegetables in the shrimp stock until tender, about 3 to 5 minutes. Divide the vegetables between 4 soup bowls. Uncover the shellfish and rearrange the shellfish on the vegetables and add the basil sprigs. Sprinkle with lemon juice.

Remove the bay leaf before serving.

Makes 4 servings

NUTRITION AT A GLANCE

Per serving: 390 calories, 18 g fat, 6 g saturated fat, 28 g protein, 33 g carbohydrate, 10 g dietary fiber, 110 mg cholesterol, 740 mg sodium

Almond Perch Sauté

This sautéed perch goes so well with the wonderfully nutty flavor of almonds.

> 1 cup 1% milk
>
> 1 egg, beaten
>
> 1 1/2 cups sliced mushrooms
>
> 1/2 cup chopped hickory smoke–flavored almonds
>
> 3 tablespoons + 3 tablespoons extra virgin olive oil
>
> 2 tablespoons chopped parsley
>
> 1 tablespoon lemon juice
>
> 2 pounds perch or grouper fillets

In a small bowl, whisk together the milk and egg. In a large bowl, combine the mushrooms, almonds, the 3 tablespoons oil, parsley, and lemon juice.

Preheat the oven to 400°F.

Heat the remaining 1/4 cup oil in a large nonstick skillet over medium heat.

Dip the fish in the egg mixture. Place the fish in one of the skillets and cook for 3 to 5 minutes, or until golden brown. Turn the fish, place in a nonstick baking dish, and bake for 5 minutes. Wipe the skillet clean. Add the almond mixture to the skillet while the fish is in the oven and cook, stirring frequently, for 5 minutes.

To serve, place the fish on a serving platter and spoon the almond mixture over the fish.

Makes 4 servings

NUTRITION AT A GLANCE

Per serving: 270 calories, 18 g fat, 2 1/2 g saturated fat, 25 g protein, 4 g carbohydrate, 1 g dietary fiber, 75 mg cholesterol, 130 mg sodium

Cod with Peppercorns and Leeks

Cracked pepper gives a nice bite to mild cod fillets, while leeks sautéed with garlic and lemon are the perfect accompaniment.

1/2	teaspoon black peppercorns, freshly cracked
1/2	teaspoon fennel seeds, finely crushed
4	fillets cod (5 ounces each)
1	tablespoon extra virgin olive oil
3	medium leeks, white part only, thinly sliced
3	scallions, finely chopped
2	cloves garlic, minced
2	teaspoons whole wheat flour
1/4	cup white wine
1/4	cup chicken broth
2	tablespoons 1% milk

Heat oven to 375°F.

Press the peppercorns and fennel seeds into both sides of the fillets. Set aside.

Heat the oil in an ovenproof skillet over medium heat. Add the leeks, scallions, and garlic and cook, stirring frequently, for 4 minutes, or until tender. Stir in the flour and cook for 1 minute. Stir in the wine, broth, and milk and bring to a boil. Remove from the heat.

Place the fish on top of the leek mixture in the skillet and bake for 10 minutes, or until the fish flakes easily. Serve the fish topped with the leek mixture.

Makes 4 servings

NUTRITION AT A GLANCE

Per serving: 203 calories, 5 g fat, 1 g saturated fat, 27 g protein, 10 g carbohydrate, 2 g dietary fiber, 61 mg cholesterol, 157 mg sodium

From the Menu of . . .

LE BERNARDIN

787 Seventh Avenue, New York City

CHEF ERIC RIPERT

LE BERNARDIN IS NEW YORK CITY'S FINEST SEAFOOD
RESTAURANT AND RENOWNED CHEF ERIC RIPERT
IS A PARTICIPANT IN THE ANNUAL
SOUTH BEACH WINE AND FOOD FESTIVAL.

Grouper with Baby Bok Choy and Soy-Ginger Vinaigrette

PHASE 3

12	heads baby bok choy (about 2 pounds)
	Salt
1	tablespoon finely diced ginger
2	tablespoons finely diced shallots
1	tablespoon oyster sauce
2	tablespoons sherry vinegar
4	tablespoons canola oil
1	tablespoon light soy sauce
1/2	teaspoon fresh lime juice

Small pinch ground red pepper

1/4 cup water

2 tablespoons unsalted butter

Fine sea salt

Freshly ground white pepper

2 tablespoons canola oil

4 grouper fillets (7-ounces each)

1 tablespoon toasted sesame seeds

Bring a large pot of water to a boil. Trim off the root ends of the bok choy, separate the leaves, and wash them well. Salt the water and add the bok choy. Blanch until just tender, about 1 1/2 minutes. Immediately plunge the bok choy into a bowl of ice water until cool. Drain and set aside.

Put the ginger and shallots in a mixing bowl and whisk in the oyster sauce and vinegar. Whisk in 4 tablespoons of canola oil, the soy sauce, lime juice, and red pepper. Set aside.

Bring the 1/4 cup of water to a boil in a large saucepan over high heat. Whisk in the butter and lower the heat to medium-high. Season the bok choy with salt and pepper, add it to the pan, and cook until heated through, about 2 minutes.

Meanwhile, divide the 2 tablespoon of canola between two 10" nonstick skillets. Place over high heat until the oil is just smoking. Season both sides of the grouper with salt and pepper. Place 2 grouper fillets in each skillet and sauté until the fish is browned on the bottom, about 3 minutes. Turn and sauté about 3 minutes more, until the fish flakes easily with a fork.

Lift the bok choy out of the pan with a slotted spoon and arrange it in the center of four dinner plates. Top with the grouper. Whisk the sauce lightly and spoon it around the bok choy. Sprinkle the sesame seeds over the sauce and serve immediately.

Makes 4 servings

NUTRITION AT A GLANCE

Per serving: 470 calories, 30 g fat, 6 g saturated fat, 42 g protein, 7 g carbohydrate, 2 g dietary fiber, 90 mg cholesterol, 440 mg sodium

Seafood-Stuffed Sole

Don't be put off by the number of ingredients here. This elegant dish is quick to assemble and can easily be prepared ahead.

Stuffed Sole

- 1 teaspoon extra virgin olive oil
- 2 cloves garlic, minced
- 1/2 cup chopped fennel
- 4 scallions, chopped
- 2 tablespoons chopped Italian parsley
- 1 1/2 teaspoons dried basil
- 3 tablespoons chopped shallots
- 8 ounces large shrimp, peeled, deveined, and sliced into thirds
- 4 ounces bay scallops
- 1 cup fresh whole wheat bread crumbs
- 1 egg, beaten
- 1 tablespoon lemon juice
- Ground black pepper
- 4 fillets sole (6 ounces each)
- 1 cup white wine

Saffron Sauce

- 1 teaspoon extra virgin olive oil
- 1 clove garlic, minced
- 1/8 teaspoon saffron threads, crushed

2 tablespoons hot water

1/2 teaspoon Dijon mustard

1/2 teaspoon capers, rinsed and drained

1 tablespoon fat-free sour cream

Salt

Ground black pepper

1 tablespoon chopped Italian parsley (optional)

To make the stuffed sole: Preheat the oven to 400°F.

Heat the oil in a large nonstick skillet over medium heat. Add the garlic, fennel, scallions, parsley, basil, and 2 tablespoons of the shallots. Cook for 4 minutes, or until the fennel is just tender. Add the shrimp and scallops and cook for 2 minutes, or until the shrimp and scallops are opaque and cooked through.

Remove the mixture to a large bowl and stir in the bread crumbs, egg, and lemon juice. Season with the pepper.

Place the sole, skin side up, on a work surface. Divide the stuffing into 4 equal portions. Slightly mound the stuffing in the center of each fillet and roll up the fillets jelly-roll style.

Coat a 1-quart baking dish with cooking spray. Sprinkle the dish with the remaining 1 tablespoon shallots and place the fillets, seam sides down, on top of the shallots. Pour the wine around the fillets. Cover with a piece of waxed paper.

Bake for 15 minutes, or until the fish is opaque and flakes easily. Remove from the baking dish and keep warm on a covered serving platter. Reserve the cooking liquid.

To make the saffron sauce: Heat the oil in a small nonstick skillet over medium heat. Add the garlic and cook for 1 minute. In a cup, mix the saffron with the water and add to the skillet. Stir in the mustard, capers, and the reserved fish-cooking liquid. Cook until the liquid is reduced to about 2/3 cup. Remove from the heat and whisk in the sour cream. Season with the salt and pepper. Spoon the sauce over the fillets and sprinkle with the parsley, if using.

Makes 4 servings

NUTRITION AT A GLANCE
Per serving: 373 calories, 8 g fat, 2 g saturated fat, 52 g protein, 11 g carbohydrate, 2 g dietary fiber, 248 mg cholesterol, 369 mg sodium

From the Menu of . . .
SMITH & WOLLENSKY
1 Washington Avenue, Miami Beach

CHEF ROBERT MIGNOLA

Smith & Wollensky is known as a great steakhouse across the country, but this salad shows there's something for everyone on the menu.

Asparagus, Crabmeat, and Grapefruit Salad
PHASE 2

Salad

- 12 pieces jumbo asparagus, trimmed stems, peeled 3" at base, steamed until just cooked, but still bright green and crisp and chilled
- 2 cups mixed baby greens
- 1/2 pound colossal lump crabmeat, picked over for bits of shell
- 12 pieces of grapefruit sections
- 1 red bell pepper, chopped

1/2 cup Citrus Vinaigrette (recipe following)

2 tablespoons minced chives

Citrus Vinaigrette

1 teaspoon Dijon mustard

1 tablespoon lemon juice

1 tablespoon lime juice

1 tablespoon orange juice

1/3 cup extra virgin olive oil

Salt

Pepper

To make the salad: Lay 3 asparagus on each plate.

Put 1/2 cup greens on top of the asparagus on each plate to make a bed for the crabmeat. Divide the crabmeat evenly into 4 portions and place it on top of the greens. Arrange the grapefruit sections around the crabmeat. Sprinkle with the bell pepper.

Drizzle with Citrus Vinaigrette. Sprinkle on chives.

To make the Citrus Vinaigrette: In a small glass or stainless steel bowl, combine the mustard, lemon juice, lime juice, and orange juice. Slowly whisk in the oil. Season with salt and pepper to taste.

Makes 4 servings

NUTRITION AT A GLANCE

Per serving: 260 calories, 20 g fat, 3 g saturated fat, 13 g protein, 9 g carbohydrate, 0 g dietary fiber, 30 mg cholesterol, 490 mg sodium

Big Easy Shrimp

Here's a quicker way to enjoy the traditional shrimp Creole dish. Serve over hot cooked brown rice for a quick Phase 2 dinner. If you like, you can substitute sea scallops for the shrimp.

2	strips turkey bacon or Canadian bacon
1	onion, chopped
1/2	green bell pepper, chopped
1	rib celery, chopped
1	clove garlic, minced
1	can (16 ounces) chopped tomatoes
1	bay leaf
1/2	teaspoon ground black pepper
1	teaspoon Worcestershire sauce
1	teaspoon hot-pepper sauce
1	pound medium shrimp, peeled and deveined

Cook the bacon in a large skillet over medium heat until crisp. Place on a paper towel–lined plate to drain. Crumble when cool. Remove and discard all but 1 tablespoon drippings from the skillet.

In the hot drippings over medium heat, cook the onion, bell pepper, and celery for 5 minutes, or until tender. Stir in the garlic and cook for 1 minute. Add the tomatoes (with juice), bay leaf, black pepper, Worcestershire sauce, and hot-pepper sauce. Heat to boiling. Reduce the heat to low and simmer for

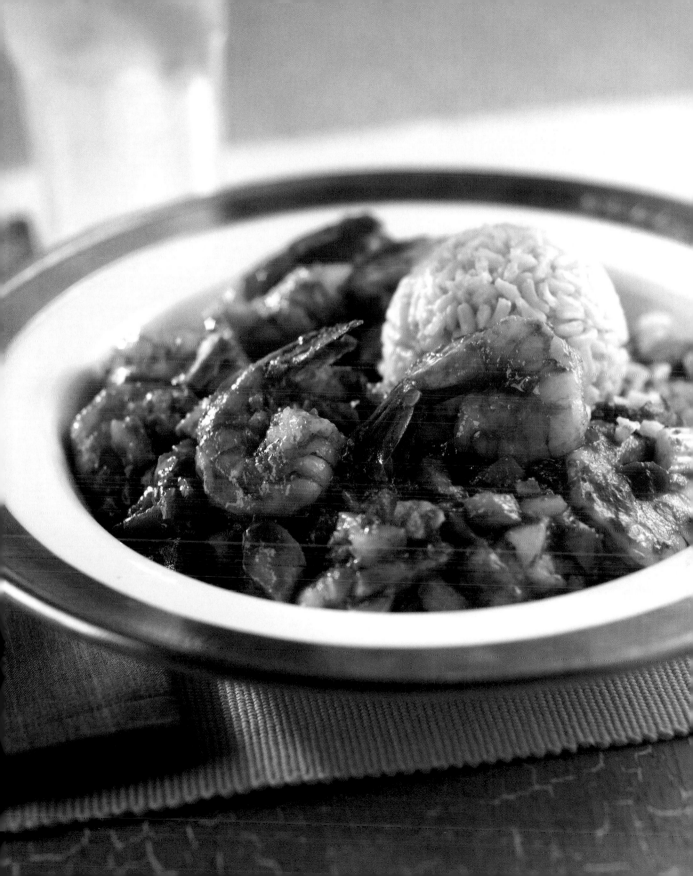

20 minutes. Add the shrimp and bacon and cook for 10 minutes, or until the shrimp are opaque. Remove and discard the bay leaf before serving.

Makes 4 servings

NUTRITION AT A GLANCE

Per serving: 185 calories, 4 g fat, 1 g saturated fat, 26 g protein, 12 g carbohydrate, 3 g dietary fiber, 177 mg cholesterol, 329 mg sodium

Caribbean Baked Chicken with Mango

All the traditional spices of Jamaican Jerk–style cookery are used in this recipe. Bake up this chicken in Phase 2 for an authentic island treat.

2	jalapeño chile peppers, halved and seeded (wear plastic gloves when handling)
1/2	onion, halved
2	cloves garlic, minced
1	slice (1/4" thick) peeled fresh ginger
1	tablespoon extra virgin olive oil
1	tablespoon white wine vinegar
1	teaspoon jerk seasoning
1	teaspoon ground allspice
1/4	teaspoon salt
4	boneless, skinless chicken breast halves
1/2	mango, peeled and finely chopped
1	tablespoon chopped fresh cilantro

Preheat the oven to 450°F. Coat a 13" × 9" baking pan with cooking spray.

In a food processor, combine the peppers, onion, garlic, ginger, oil, vinegar, jerk seasoning, allspice, and salt. Process until very finely chopped, stopping the machine a few times to scrape down the sides of the container.

Spread the jalapeño mixture on both sides of the chicken breasts. Place the chicken breasts, skinned side up, in the prepared baking pan.

Bake for 30 minutes, or until a thermometer inserted in the thickest portion registers 170°F and the juices run clear.

Place the chicken on plates and scatter the mango on top. Sprinkle with the cilantro.

Makes 4 servings

NUTRITION AT A GLANCE

Per serving: 186 calories, 5 g fat, 1 g saturated fat, 28 g protein, 6 g carbohydrate, 1 g dietary fiber, 68 mg cholesterol, 264 mg sodium

Tropical Glazed Chicken

Pineapple juice and honey paired with a hint of mustard and red pepper give this dish a delightful sweet-and-spicy punch. You can make the glaze ahead, making this an easy dish for a busy weeknight.

> 1 cup chicken broth
>
> 3 tablespoons pineapple juice concentrate, thawed
>
> 1 tablespoon coarse-grain Dijon mustard
>
> 1 clove garlic, minced
>
> 1 teaspoon fincly chopped fresh sage
>
> 1/2 teaspoon mustard powder
>
> Dash of ground red pepper
>
> 1 tablespoon honey
>
> 1 pound boneless, skinless chicken breasts

Bring the chicken broth to a boil in a small saucepan over medium-high heat until it is reduced to 1/4 cup. Add the juice, mustard, garlic, sage, mustard powder, red pepper, and honey. Bring to a boil, reduce the heat to low, and simmer for 5 minutes, stirring occasionally. Remove from the heat. Use immediately or refrigerate until ready to use.

Coat a grill rack with cooking spray. Preheat the grill for 10 minutes on medium-high.

Grill the chicken for 4 minutes. Turn and grill for 1 minute longer. Brush with the pineapple–mustard glaze. Grill for 4 minutes longer, brushing with the glaze, until a thermometer inserted in the thickest portion registers 170°F and the juices run clear.

Makes 4 servings

NUTRITION AT A GLANCE

Per serving: 161 calories, 2 g fat, 1 g saturated fat, 27 g protein, 7 g carbohydrate, 0 g dietary fiber, 66 mg cholesterol, 419 mg sodium

Coconut Chicken

If Bali is the ultimate island, then this dinner is the ultimate Bali taste. Chicken braised in coconut milk (Opor Ayam) is a true classic of Indonesian fare. We did change the chicken to white meat instead of the traditional drumstick or wing. New traditions can sometimes be better than old ones.

2 tablespoons extra virgin olive oil

1 pound chicken breast tenders

1 tablespoon chicken broth

1 medium onion, chopped

2 cloves garlic, minced

3/4 teaspoon dried cilantro

1 teaspoon grated fresh ginger

1 teaspoon finely grated lemon peel

1/8 teaspoon ground cumin

Pinch of ground turmeric

1 cup light coconut milk (no sugar added)

2 tablespoons macadamia nuts, finely ground

1 teaspoon sugar substitute

1/4 teaspoon ground red pepper

1 tablespoon tamarind paste (available in Indian and specialty food markets)

2 teaspoons water

Chopped scallion, for garnish

Heat the oil in a large skillet over medium-high heat. Add the chicken and cook for 5 minutes per side, or until browned and no longer pink in the center. Remove the chicken to a plate and set aside.

Heat the broth in the same skillet. Add the onion, garlic, cilantro, ginger, lemon peel, cumin, and turmeric and cook for 5 minutes, or until the onion is

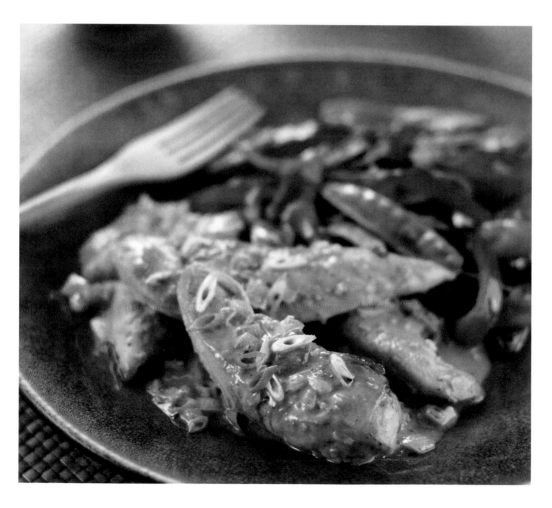

tender but not browned. Stir in the coconut milk, nuts, sugar substitute, and red pepper. Return the chicken to the skillet, cover, and simmer for 10 minutes, or until the chicken is cooked through.

Remove the chicken to a plate and keep warm. Do not discard the sauce in the pan.

In a small bowl, combine the tamarind paste and water. Stir into the sauce in the skillet and gently boil until thickened and the mixture measures about 1 cup.

Evenly divide the chicken among 4 serving plates. Top with sauce and garnish with the scallion.

Makes 4 servings

NUTRITION AT A GLANCE

Per serving: 360 calories, 25 g fat, 14 g saturated fat, 28 g protein, 10 g carbohydrate, 3 g dietary fiber, 66 mg cholesterol, 60 mg sodium

Chicken with Lime Dressing

This Tex-Mex-styled chicken is sure to be a favorite. It will turn your home into a hacienda for the evening.

Lime Dressing

- 1/3 cup fresh lime juice
- 1/4 cup chopped fresh cilantro
- 1 tablespoon chopped scallions
- 1 tablespoon extra virgin olive oil
- 1 teaspoon sugar substitute
- 1/2 teaspoon salt

Chicken

- 4 boneless, skinless chicken breast halves, pounded to 1/2" thickness
- 2 medium avocados, peeled and pitted
- 1 tablespoon fresh lemon juice
- 2 teaspoons picante sauce
- 1 teaspoon + 1 tablespoon extra virgin olive oil
- 1 medium red bell pepper, finely chopped
- 1 clove garlic, minced
- 1/4 cup sliced almonds, toasted
- 2 tablespoons whole wheat flour

To make the dressing: In a large bowl, combine the lime juice, cilantro, scallions, oil, sugar substitute, and salt.

To make the chicken: In a large glass dish, combine the

chicken with 3 tablespoons of the lime dressing. Cover and refrigerate for 10 minutes.

In a medium bowl, mash the avocados with 2 tablespoons of the lime dressing. Stir in the lemon juice and picante sauce. Reserve the remaining lime dressing.

Heat 1 teaspoon of the oil in a large nonstick skillet. Add the pepper and cook, stirring occasionally, for 6 minutes, or until the pepper is tender and lightly browned. Stir in the garlic and cook for 30 seconds. Remove to a large bowl and add the almonds.

Remove the chicken from the dressing and pat dry with paper towels. Sprinkle flour over both sides of the chicken.

Heat the remaining 1 tablespoon oil in a large skillet over medium-high heat. Add the chicken and cook for 6 minutes on each side, or until a thermometer inserted in the thickest portion registers 170°F and the juices run clear. Place the chicken on 4 serving plates and equally divide the pepper mixture, sprinkling over the chicken. Drizzle the reserved dressing over each serving. Serve with a side of the mashed avocados.

Makes 4 servings

NUTRITION AT A GLANCE

Per serving: 429 calories, 27 g fat, 4 g saturated fat, 33 g protein, 19 g carbohydrate, 10 g dietary fiber, 68 mg cholesterol, 382 mg sodium

From the Menu of . . .
BOLO RESTAURANT & BAR
23 E. 22nd Street, New York City

CHEF BOBBY FLAY

BOBBY FLAY IS ANOTHER GREAT CHEF WHO TAKES PART IN THE SOUTH BEACH WINE AND FOOD FESTIVAL. HIS RESTAURANTS IN NEW YORK ARE ALWAYS HOPPIN'.

Spanish Spiced Rubbed Chicken with Mustard-Green Onion Sauce

PHASE 1

Mustard-Green Onion Sauce

- 1/2 cup aged white wine vinegar
- 3 tablespoons Dijon mustard
- 1 cup extra virgin olive oil

    Salt

    Freshly ground black pepper

- 1/2 cup thinly sliced scallions
- 3 tablespoons finely chopped flat-leaf parsley

Spanish Spice Rub

- 3 tablespoons Spanish or regular paprika
- 1 tablespoon cumin seeds, ground
- 1 tablespoon mustard seeds, ground
- 2 teaspoons fennel seeds, ground
- 2 teaspoons coarsely ground black pepper
- 2 teaspoons kosher salt

Chicken

- 8 bone-in chicken breasts, French cut

Extra virgin olive oil

Salt

Spanish Spice Rub (above)

Chopped parsley, for garnish

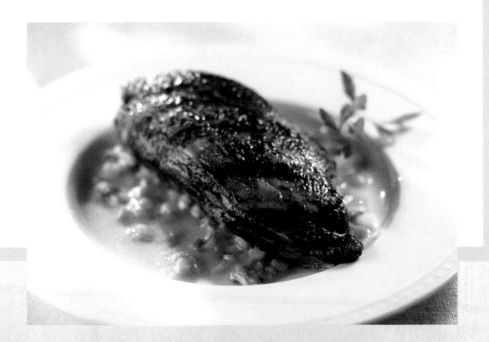

To make the sauce: In a large bowl, whisk together the vinegar and mustard. Slowly whisk in the oil until emulsified (well combined) and season with salt and pepper to taste. Fold in the scallions and parsley.

To make the spice rub: In a small bowl, whisk together the paprika, cumin, mustard seeds, fennel seeds, pepper, and salt, and set aside.

To make the chicken: Heat the grill to medium. Brush the chicken breasts with olive oil. Season each chicken breast with salt on both sides. Rub each chicken breast on the skin side with the spice rub and place on the grill, rub-side down. Grill for 5 to 6 minutes or until slightly charred and a crust has formed. Turn the chicken breasts over, close the cover, and continue cooking for 6 to 7 minutes or until just cooked through. Spoon some of the Mustard–Green Onion Sauce onto a platter and place the chicken breasts on top. Garnish with chopped parsley and serve the remaining sauce on the side.

Note: French cut means to make a cut along the chicken bone, exposing the flesh.

Makes 8 servings

NUTRITION AT A GLANCE

Per serving: 357 calories, 24 g fat, 4 g saturated fat, 19 g protein, 5 g carbohydrate, 2 g dietary fiber, 43 mg cholesterol, 779 mg sodium

Chicken Mole

This delicious, spicy chicken will be perfect any time for you chocolate lovers out there.

2 1/2	pounds chicken breast tenders
	Salt
	Ground black pepper
1	large onion, chopped
1	large green bell pepper, cored, seeded, and chopped
2	cloves garlic, minced
2	tablespoons chili powder
1/2	teaspoon ground cinnamon
1/2	teaspoon ground cloves
1	can (14 1/2 ounces) diced tomatoes
2	tablespoons unsweetened natural peanut butter
2	tablespoons unsweetened cocoa powder
2	scallions, chopped

Sprinkle the chicken with salt and black pepper. Heat a large nonstick skillet coated with olive oil cooking spray over medium-high heat. Add the chicken and cook for 8 minutes, turning once, or until browned on both sides. Remove the chicken to a large plate.

Add the onion, bell pepper, and garlic to the skillet and cook for 3 minutes, or until the onion becomes translucent. Stir in the chili powder, cinnamon, and cloves and cook for 1 minute. Return the chicken to the skillet. Add the tomatoes (with juice), peanut butter, and cocoa powder and bring to a boil. Cover and simmer, stirring every few minutes, for 25 minutes, turning once, or until the chicken is no longer pink. Garnish with the scallions.

Makes 4 servings

NUTRITION AT A GLANCE

Per serving: 431 calories, 8 g fat, 2 g saturated fat, 70 g protein, 17 g carbohydrate, 6 g dietary fiber, 164 mg cholesterol, 398 mg sodium

Artichoke Chicken

Every vegetable has its holiday, and March 16 is National Artichoke Day. But you could serve this any day!

- 4 tablespoons extra virgin olive oil
- 4 boneless, skinless chicken breast halves, pounded to 1/2" thickness
- 1 bag (16 ounces) frozen small whole onions
- 1 can (13 3/4 ounces) chicken broth
- 1 tablespoon balsamic vinegar
- Salt
- Ground black pepper
- 1 package (10 ounces) frozen artichoke hearts

Heat 2 tablespoons of the oil in a large skillet over medium heat. Add the chicken and cook for 10 minutes, turning once, or until browned on both sides. Carefully remove the chicken to a large bowl.

Heat the remaining 2 tablespoons oil in the skillet. Add the onions and cook, stirring occasionally, for 5 minutes, or until lightly browned. Return the chicken to the pan and add the chicken broth and vinegar, and season with salt and pepper. Bring to a boil. Reduce the heat to low, cover, and simmer for 20 minutes. Add the artichoke hearts and cook for 10 minutes, or until the artichokes are tender and a thermometer inserted in the thickest portion of a chicken breast registers 170°F and the juices run clear.

Makes 4 servings

NUTRITION AT A GLANCE

Per serving: 337 calories, 16 g fat, 2 g saturated fat, 32 g protein, 17 g carbohydrate, 7 g dietary fiber, 68 mg cholesterol, 529 mg sodium

Spice-Rubbed Chicken Fingers with Cilantro Dipping Sauce

This cool green dipping sauce is the perfect accompaniment, but if you prefer, you can substitute prepared sugar-free barbecue sauce.

1	teaspoon chili powder
1	teaspoon ground cumin
1/4	teaspoon salt
1	pound chicken breast tenders
1/2	cup cilantro sprigs
1/4	cup parsley sprigs
1/4	cup blanched slivered almonds
1	clove garlic
1	serrano chile pepper, seeded (wear plastic gloves when handling)
1/8	teaspoon salt
2	tablespoons lime juice
2	tablespoons extra virgin olive oil
2	tablespoons water
	Sprig cilantro, for garnish

Coat a grill rack or broiler-pan rack with cooking spray. Preheat the grill or broiler.

In a cup, combine the chili powder, cumin, and salt. Cut two 1/2"-deep slashes in each side of the chicken tenders. Rub the spice mixture over the chicken, pressing it into the slits. Place the chicken in a baking pan and coat completely with cooking spray. Let stand for 10 minutes.

In a food processor, combine the cilantro, parsley, almonds, garlic, chile pepper, and salt. Process until chopped. While the processor is running, add the lime juice and oil through the feed tube, stopping the machine once or twice to scrape down the sides of the container until the sauce is smooth. Pour the sauce into a bowl. Stir in the water, cover, and chill until ready to serve.

Place the chicken on the prepared rack and grill or broil 6" from the heat, turning several times, for 15 minutes, or until a thermometer inserted in the thickest portion registers 170°F and the juices run clear. Serve with the sauce and garnish with the cilantro.

Makes 4 servings

NUTRITION AT A GLANCE
Per serving: 248 calories, 13 g fat, 2 g saturated fat, 28 g protein, 4 g carbohydrate, 1 g dietary fiber, 66 mg cholesterol, 324 mg sodium

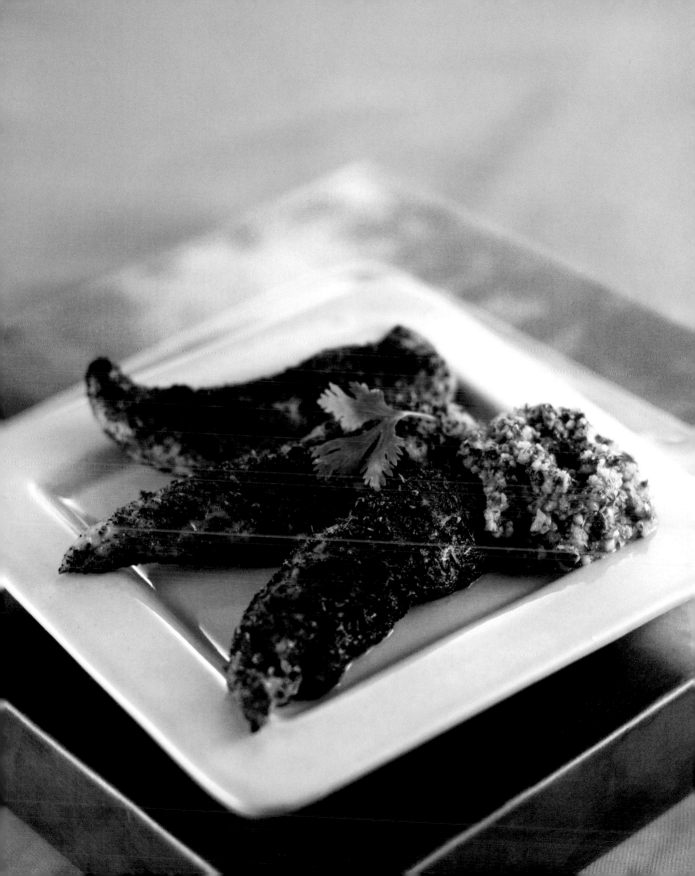

Chicken Capri

This dish tastes like it took you all day, but it can be done in 30 minutes. The chicken goes especially well with a crisp garden salad topped with any South Beach–approved dressing.

- 1 cup reduced-fat ricotta cheese
- 1/2 teaspoon dried oregano
- 1/4 teaspoon salt
- 1/4 teaspoon ground black pepper
- 4 boneless, skinless chicken breast halves
- 1/2 teaspoon garlic powder
- 2 tablespoons extra virgin olive oil
- 1 cup crushed tomatoes
- 4 slices reduced-fat mozzarella cheese

In a blender or food processor, combine the ricotta with the oregano, salt, and pepper. Process to blend.

Rub the chicken with the garlic powder. Heat the oil in a large skillet over medium-high heat. Add the chicken and cook for 12 minutes per side. Place the chicken breasts, side by side, in a large baking dish and allow to cool.

Preheat the oven to 350°F.

Spoon 1/4 cup of the cheese mixture and 1/4 cup tomatoes onto each chicken breast. Top each chicken breast with 1 slice mozzarella. Bake for 20 minutes, or until a thermometer inserted in the thickest portion of a breast registers 170°F and the juices run clear.

Makes 4 servings

NUTRITION AT A GLANCE
Per serving: 340 calories, 15 g fat, 5 g saturated fat, 44 g protein, 6 g carbohydrate, 1 g dietary fiber, 115 mg cholesterol, 470 mg sodium

Spicy Chinese Chicken Kebabs

These sensational skewers are excellent served chilled or warm. Serve them with hot brown rice and a side salad of fresh baby greens to round out the meal.

- 2 tablespoons orange juice
- 1 1/2 tablespoons hoisin sauce
- 1 tablespoon South Beach Ketchup (see page 242) or sugar-free ketchup
- 1 tablespoon rice vinegar
- 1 tablespoon prepared Chinese chili sauce with garlic
- 1 teaspoon light soy sauce
- 1 teaspoon toasted sesame oil
- 1 teaspoon grated orange peel
- 1 1/2 pounds boneless, skinless chicken breasts, cut into 1" pieces

In a 1-quart zip-top plastic bag, combine the orange juice, hoisin sauce, ketchup, vinegar, chili sauce, soy sauce, oil, and orange peel. Add the chicken. Seal the bag securely and turn to coat the chicken. Refrigerate the chicken for at least 2 hours, turning the bag occasionally.

Coat a grill rack or broiler-pan rack with cooking spray. Preheat the grill or broiler.

Thread the chicken pieces onto 6 metal skewers. Place the skewers on the prepared rack and grill over hot coals for 5 minutes per side, or until the chicken is no longer pink. Or broil 4 inches from the heat for 7 minutes per side, or until a thermometer inserted in the thickest portion registers 170° and the juices run clear.

Makes 6 servings

NUTRITION AT A GLANCE

Per serving: 150 calories, 2 g fat, 1 g saturated fat, 26 g protein, 4 g carbohydrate, 0 g dietary fiber, 66 mg cholesterol, 282 mg sodium

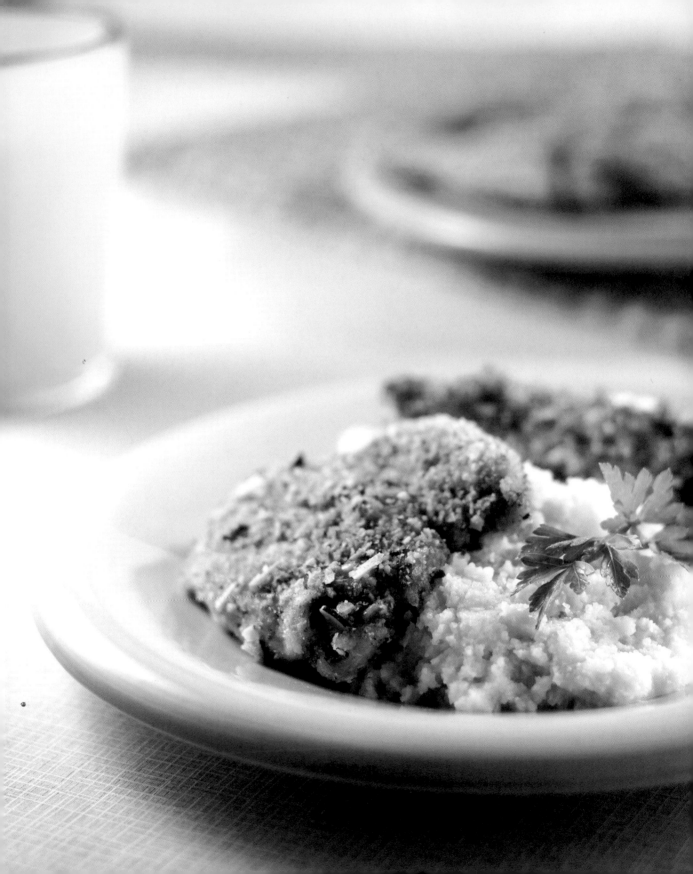

Oven-Fried Chicken with Almonds

You don't have to fry your chicken to get that fried taste. This recipe is cooked in the oven and has a faint nuttiness from the almonds to top it off.

1	cup whole wheat bread crumbs
1/4	cup (1 ounce) grated Parmesan cheese
1/4	cup finely chopped almonds
2	tablespoons chopped parsley
1	clove garlic, crushed
1	teaspoon salt
1/4	teaspoon dried thyme
	Pinch of ground black pepper
1/4	cup extra virgin olive oil
2	pounds boneless, skinless chicken breasts, pounded to 1/2" thickness and cut into 12 pieces
	Sprig Italian parsley, for garnish

Preheat the oven to 400°F.

In a medium bowl, combine the bread crumbs, cheese, almonds, parsley, garlic, salt, thyme, and pepper. Mix thoroughly.

Place the oil in a shallow dish. Dip the chicken first in the oil, then dredge in the crumb mixture. Place the chicken in a shallow baking pan.

Bake for 25 minutes, or until a thermometer inserted in the center of a piece registers 170°F and the juices run clear. (Do not turn the chicken during cooking.) Garnish with the parsley.

Makes 6 servings

NUTRITION AT A GLANCE

Per serving: 383 calories, 16 g fat, 4 g saturated fat, 41 g protein, 15 g carbohydrate, 1 g dietary fiber, 91 mg cholesterol, 730 mg sodium

Five-Spice Chicken

Ginger, soy, and Chinese five-spice powder give this spicy dinner its Asian flair. If this is your first experience with five-spice powder, you may want to reduce the amount by half in this recipe to give the dish a little less heat.

- 3 tablespoons dry sherry
- 2 tablespoons light soy sauce
- 1 tablespoon brown-sugar-substitute syrup or 2 tablespoons granulated brown sugar substitute (see note)
- 1 teaspoon finely chopped fresh ginger
- 1 clove garlic, minced
- 1/2 teaspoon Chinese five-spice powder
- 4 boneless, skinless chicken breast halves
- 1 teaspoon cornstarch
- 1 tablespoon cold water
- 2 scallions, thinly sliced, for garnish

In a shallow 1 1/2-quart microwaveable dish, combine the sherry, soy sauce, sugar substitute brown sugar syrup, ginger, garlic, and five-spice powder. Add the chicken and turn to coat. Cover with vented plastic wrap and microwave for 5 minutes on high power. Turn the chicken and cook for 5 minutes longer, or until a thermometer inserted in the thickest portion of a breast registers 170°F and the juices run clear. Place the chicken on a serving platter. Do not discard the juices in the dish.

In a cup, dissolve the cornstarch in the water and stir into the juices in the dish. Cover with vented plastic wrap and microwave on high power for 1 1/2 minutes. Stir and pour over the chicken. Sprinkle the scallions over the top for garnish.

Note: Splenda brown sugar syrup is available at www.naturesflavors.com and Sugar Twin brown sugar replacement is available in stores and at www.lowcarb.com.

Makes 4 servings

NUTRITION AT A GLANCE

Per serving: 165 calories, 2 g fat, 0 g saturated fat, 28 g protein, 6 g carbohydrate, 0 g dietary fiber, 68 mg cholesterol, 384 mg sodium

Ginger Chicken

The slightly hot, citruslike taste and wonderful aroma from the ginger makes for a true delight when blended with the teriyaki sauce.

> 1 piece (6 inches) fresh ginger, peeled and cut into 1" pieces
>
> 2 cloves garlic
>
> 2 tablespoons extra virgin olive oil
>
> 1/2 cup South Beach Teriyaki Sauce (see page 241)
>
> 2–3 pounds chicken breasts on the bone
>
> Salt
>
> Ground black pepper

Preheat the oven to 450°F.

In a blender or food processor, combine the ginger, garlic, and oil. Process until finely chopped. While the machine is running, add the teriyaki sauce until the mixture has a mustard-like texture.

Place the chicken in a large, shallow bowl and cover it with the ginger mixture. Cover and refrigerate for 10 minutes.

Place the chicken on a broiler pan and season with the salt and pepper. Bake until the chicken is cooked through, about 20 minutes. Lower oven to 350°F. Bake for 25 more minutes, or until a thermometer inserted in the thickest portion registers 170° to 175°F and the juices run clear.

Makes 4 servings

NUTRITION AT A GLANCE

Per serving: 468 calories, 11 g fat, 2 g saturated fat, 61 g protein, 7 g carbohydrate, 0 g dietary fiber, 197 mg cholesterol, 862 mg sodium

Sesame Baked Chicken

The mild, nutty flavor from the sesame seeds provides just the right lift to this chicken.

   1 egg, lightly beaten
   2 tablespoons canola oil
   1 teaspoon toasted sesame oil
   1 tablespoon water
   1 tablespoon light soy sauce
1/2 teaspoon salt
1/4 teaspoon ground black pepper
   2 tablespoons uncooked oat bran
1/4 cup sesame seeds
1 1/2 pounds boneless, skinless chicken breasts, cut into 2" pieces

Preheat the oven to 350°F.

In a shallow bowl, combine the egg, canola oil, sesame oil, water, soy sauce, salt, and pepper.

In a small bowl, combine the oat bran and sesame seeds.

Dip the chicken in the egg mixture, then dredge in the bran mixture. Place the chicken in a 11" × 7" nonstick baking pan.

Bake for 30 minutes, or until the chicken is no longer pink in the center and a thermometer inserted in the center of a piece registers 170°F and the juices run clear.

Makes 4 servings

NUTRITION AT A GLANCE

Per serving: 339 calories, 16 g fat, 2 g saturated fat, 43 g protein, 5 g carbohydrate, 2 g dietary fiber, 152 mg cholesterol, 568 mg sodium

Grilled Raspberry Chicken

This recipe offers down-home and delicious summer flavor! Although you can use frozen berries, fresh taste best. Use your own homegrown berries or buy them at a local market.

1/2	cup raspberry vinegar
1/2	cup red wine
1/4	cup Worcestershire sauce
4	cloves garlic, minced
1	teaspoon black pepper
2	pounds boneless, skinless chicken breasts
4	cups cooked brown and wild rice pilaf
	Sprigs of watercress or parsley, for garnish
	Fresh or frozen raspberries (without syrup and thawed, if frozen), for garnish

In a large glass baking dish, combine the vinegar, wine, Worcestershire sauce, garlic, and pepper. Place the chicken in the dish, turning to coat both sides. Cover and refrigerate for 1 hour, turning the chicken after 30 minutes.

Coat a grill rack with cooking spray. Preheat the grill.

Grill the chicken over medium-hot heat, turning halfway through and brushing frequently with the marinade, for 15 minutes, or until a thermometer inserted in the thickest portion registers 160°F and the juices run clear.

Arrange the chicken on the hot pilaf on a serving platter and garnish with the watercress or parsley and raspberries.

Makes 8 servings

NUTRITION AT A GLANCE

Per serving: 280 calories, 5 g fat, 1 g saturated fat, 29 g protein, 26 g carbohydrate, 1 g dietary fiber, 66 mg cholesterol, 234 mg sodium

Chicken and Eggplant Casserole

Chicken mixed with hearty vegetables and a hint of delicious cheese makes a glorious combination in this casserole. Make this dish ahead and cook it the next day, or make two batches and freeze one for an easy meal another day.

- 1 eggplant, peeled and cut into 12 slices
- 2 tablespoons shredded Parmesan or Asiago cheese
- 1/2 teaspoon garlic powder or 1 clove garlic, minced
- 3/4 pound boneless, skinless chicken breast, chopped
- 1 can (14 1/2 ounces) diced tomatoes
- 1 medium onion, chopped
- 1 large green bell pepper, chopped
- 1/2 cup mushrooms, sliced
- 3/4 teaspoon dried Italian seasoning
- 1/4 teaspoon ground black pepper
- 1/4 cup (1 ounce) shredded reduced-fat mozzarella cheese

Preheat the broiler.

Arrange the eggplant slices in a single layer on a nonstick baking sheet. Mist the slices with cooking spray. Broil 4 inches from the heat for 2 minutes, or until golden. Turn the eggplant over and mist again. Sprinkle with the Parmesan or Asiago cheese and garlic. Broil for 1 minute, or until golden. Set aside.

Heat a nonstick skillet coated with cooking spray over medium-high heat for 1 minute. Add the chicken and cook, stirring often, for 5 minutes, or until no longer pink. Add the tomatoes (with juice), onion, bell pepper, mushrooms, Italian seasoning, and black pepper, stirring to break up the tomatoes. Bring to a boil. Reduce the heat to low and simmer for 5 minutes.

Preheat the oven to 375°F.

Coat an 8" baking dish with cooking spray. Arrange 6 eggplant slices in the bottom of the dish. Top with the chicken mixture. Arrange the remaining 6 eggplant slices over the chicken. Sprinkle with the mozzarella cheese. Cover with foil and finish cooking, or refrigerate until the next day. Or wrap with foil, label, and freeze for up to 3 weeks.

Bake, covered, for 30 minutes, or until heated through. To cook frozen casserole, bake, covered, at 375°F for 50 minutes, or until heated through.

Makes 4 servings

NUTRITION AT A GLANCE

Per serving: 205 calories, 3 g fat, 1 g saturated fat, 26 g protein, 19 g carbohydrate, 6 g dietary fiber, 55 mg cholesterol, 395 mg sodium

From the Menu of . . .
DORAKU
1104 Lincoln Road, Miami Beach

CHEF HIROYUKI "HIRO" TERADA

DORAKU MEANS "JOY OF" IN JAPANESE, AND AT THIS LINCOLN ROAD SUSHI-AND-SAKE RESTAURANT, THERE'S PLENTY TO BE HAPPY ABOUT. THE MENU ALSO FEATURES A SELECTION OF ASIAN GRILLED DISHES.

Healthy Bird
PHASE 1

1/4 cup light soy sauce

1/4 cup water

2 cloves garlic, finely chopped

1 tablespoon chopped ginger

1 one-pound Cornish hen, quartered

2 teaspoons sesame oil

3 pieces of asparagus

In a bowl, mix the soy sauce, water, garlic, and ginger. Place the hen in the mixture and let it marinate for 1 hour.

Preheat a sauté or grill pan.

Brown the hen on all sides over medium-high heat. Place the hen in a baking dish.

Preheat the oven to 400°F.

Make a long slit through the outer skin of the hen. Baste the hen with the oil. Bake for 15 to 20 minutes, or until a thermometer inserted in the thickest portion registers 170° to 175°F and the juices run clear.

Remove the skin from the hen.

Steam the asparagus for 1 1/2 minutes until crisp.

Serve the hen with the asparagus, pouring the pan juices over the hen and asparagus.

Makes 1 serving

NUTRITION AT A GLANCE

Per serving: 400 calories, 18 g fat, 3 1/2 g saturated fat, 53 g protein, 4 g carbohydrate, 1 g dietary fiber, 235 mg cholesterol, 1,283 mg sodium

"Soufflé" Stuffed Chicken

This light and fluffy chicken recipe will fit the bill.

- 1 package (12 ounces) Stouffer's frozen spinach soufflé, not thawed
- 4 boneless, skinless chicken breasts, pounded to 1/4" thickness
- 2 tablespoons extra virgin olive oil
- 2 cloves garlic, sliced
- 1 cup chicken broth
- 2 tablespoons lemon juice
- 1 teaspoon Dijon mustard
  Salt
  Ground black pepper
- 1 tablespoon chopped parsley, for garnish
  Slices lemon, for garnish
  Sprig parsley, for garnish

Preheat the oven to 350°F.

Using a serrated knife, cut the spinach soufflé crosswise into 4 equal pieces. Top half of each whole breast with one of the pieces of soufflé. Fold half of the chicken over the filling and fasten the edges with wooden picks.

Heat the oil in a large skillet over medium-high heat. Add the garlic and cook for 3 minutes, or until golden. Discard the garlic. Add the chicken breasts to

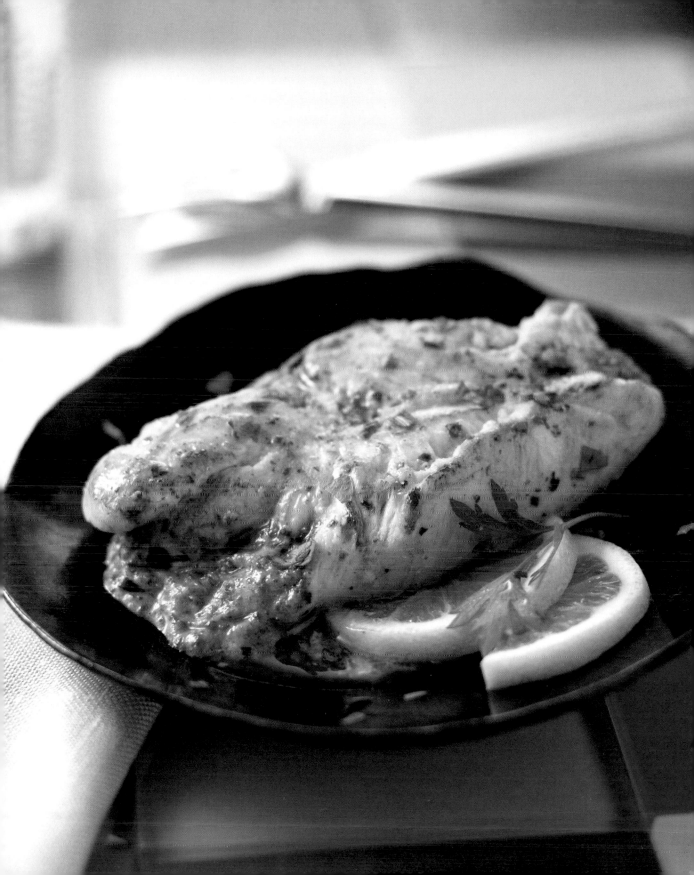

the skillet and cook for 7 minutes per side, or until well-browned on both sides.

Remove the chicken breasts to an oven-proof dish. Bake in the oven for 30 minutes, or until a thermometer inserted in the thickest portion registers 170°F and the juices run clear.

While the chicken is baking, add the broth, lemon juice, mustard, salt, and pepper to the large skillet. Heat to boiling. Reduce the heat to low, cover, and simmer for 20 minutes, or until the sauce is reduced about 1/2.

To serve, remove and discard the wooden picks. Arrange the chicken on a warm serving platter, and spoon the sauce over the chicken. Garnish with the chopped parsley, lemon, and parsley sprig.

Makes 4 servings

NUTRITION AT A GLANCE

Per serving: 308 calories, 15 g fat, 3 g saturated fat, 32 g protein, 9 g carbohydrate, 1 g dietary fiber, 136 mg cholesterol, 719 mg sodium

Creamy Chicken Paprikash

Probably one of the best-known ways to prepare chicken, this dish is deeply rooted in Eastern European tradition. If you want to use regular pasta, you can substitute it once in a while for the whole wheat for a Phase 3 dinner.

8	ounces whole wheat linguine
4	boneless, skinless chicken breast halves, cut into bite-size pieces
1/2	teaspoon salt
1/4	teaspoon ground black pepper
1	large onion, chopped
1	clove garlic, minced
3/4	cup chicken broth
2	teaspoons ground paprika
1 1/2	cups broccoli florets
1	cup fat-free sour cream

Prepare the linguine according to package directions. Drain and cover to keep warm.

Meanwhile, sprinkle the chicken with the salt and black pepper.

Heat a large nonstick skillet coated with cooking spray over medium heat. Add the chicken and cook, stirring, for 7 to 8 minutes, or until the pieces begin to brown. Remove to a plate and set aside.

Add the onion, garlic, and 3 tablespoons of the broth to the skillet. Cook, stirring, for 5 minutes, or until the onion is tender. (Add more broth if necessary to prevent sticking.)

Stir in the paprika and cook for 1 minute. Stir in the remaining broth, then add the chicken and broccoli. Bring to a boil. Reduce the heat, cover, and simmer for 20 minutes, or until the vegetables are tender.

Stir the sour cream into the chicken mixture. Cook, stirring, over low heat for 1 to 2 minutes, or until heated through. (Do not boil.) Serve the chicken over the linguine.

Makes 4 servings

NUTRITION AT A GLANCE

Per serving: 450 calories, 10 g fat, 5 g saturated fat, 39 g protein, 51 g carbohydrate, 4 g dietary fiber, 92 mg cholesterol, 301 mg sodium

Wild Rice Turkey Burgers

Almost everyone likes a good burger. If only they weren't so bad for you! This recipe is the answer to the dilemma.

1 cup wild rice

1 pound ground turkey breast

2 tablespoons South Beach Barbecue Sauce (see recipe on page 239)

1 egg, beaten

4 cubes (1" each) reduced-fat Cheddar cheese

Preheat the oven to 350°F.

Prepare the wild rice according to package directions.

In a large bowl, combine the turkey, wild rice, BBQ sauce, and egg. Divide the turkey mixture into 4 equal parts and shape into patties, placing a cube of cheese in the center of each patty.

Heat a large nonstick skillet over medium-high heat. Add the patties and sear both sides. Place the patties in a nonstick baking pan and bake for 10 minutes, or until a thermometer inserted in the center of a pattie registers 165°F and the meat is no longer pink.

Makes 4 servings

NUTRITION AT A GLANCE

Per serving: 430 calories, 15 g fat, 6 g saturated fat, 40 g protein, 31 g carbohydrate, 3 g dietary fiber, 140 mg cholesterol, 330 mg sodium

IT WAS SO ENERGIZING TO SEE THE POUNDS COMING OFF.

I started the South Beach Diet right before Thanksgiving. It was a challenge beginning right before the holidays, but I was at the point of having to either go on a diet or buy all new clothes. When I heard about the South Beach Diet, I decided to give it a try. I had no idea it would become a life plan.

I'm a sunshine, sunlight person. So for me the winter can be depressing. But after starting South Beach, I had my best winter ever. It was so energizing to see the pounds coming off. After losing the first 9 pounds in just 2 weeks, I went on to lose a total of 25. At my top weight, I was 160; now I'm 135 pounds—a comfortable size 10.

I won't say that Phase 1 was easy, because I love carbs . . . I really missed rice, bread, and pasta. But I was encouraged by losing 9 pounds right away, so that made it easier to stay away from them.

My mother had a stroke at age 60, and my dad had heart issues, so at 54, I'm pleased to be taking preventive health measures. At my last checkup, my blood work and cholesterol levels were excellent. I've also been walking three times a week, which helps me stay healthy and energized.

For breakfast, my husband and I love our omelets—a favorite is with onions, asparagus, and a little cheese. Lunch is easy—packaged green salads with some leftover protein from dinner, maybe some salmon or chicken that we've grilled the night before. My favorite snack is a Granny Smith apple with a little bit of peanut butter.

One of my favorite dinners is to top a small amount of whole wheat pasta with some low-fat turkey sausage, diced tomato, and spinach and bake it. It's great! The ricotta cheese dessert is wonderful, and sometimes we have a little sugar-free ice cream. For an extra treat, I'll shave a little dark chocolate on top of these desserts.

What I love is that you don't have to give up eating out on this plan; just learn to modify your food choices. My husband loves to try out fine restaurants. Even in Italian restaurants, I just order double vegetables instead of pasta, and I stay right on track.

It's great that I don't have those "sugar lows" any more; my energy level is more even. It's easy to enjoy being on this plan. —*SHARON L.*

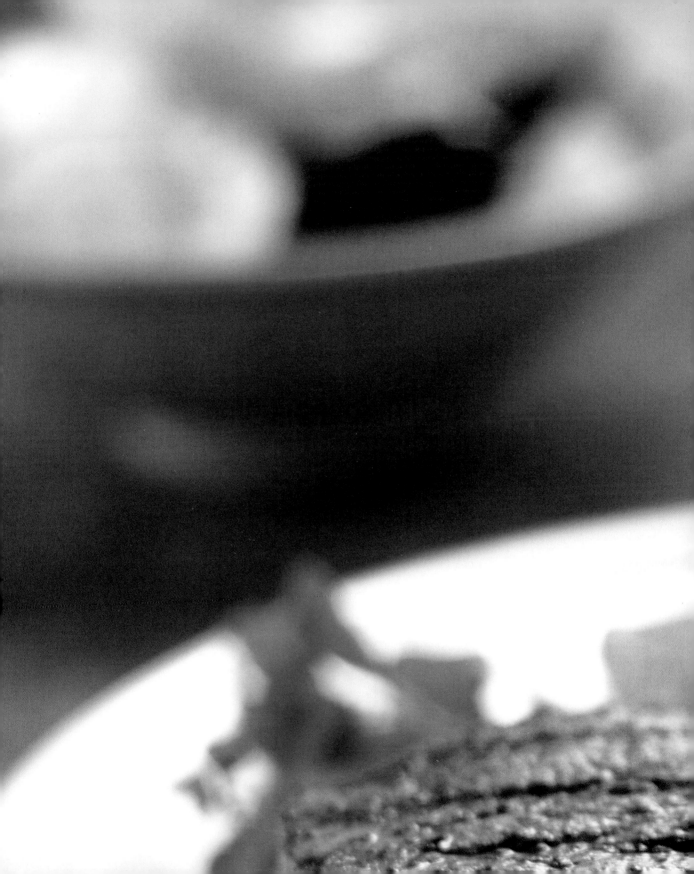

MEATS

Here is where the South Beach Diet least resembles a weight loss program. In this chapter, you'll find quite a few red-meat recipes, simply because eating beef need not be unhealthy or fattening, despite what we've all been led to believe. This is especially true if you stick with the leanest cuts—round steak (top or bottom), sirloin, round tip, tenderloin (filet mignon), or top loin. The saturated fat content in these isn't terribly high. And beef contains iron and zinc, both of which we need. Best of all, steak tastes good, and it will satisfy your hunger far better than a big plate of pasta. Be sure to steer clear of the fattiest cuts, such as brisket, prime rib, and rib eye.

And if you enjoy lamb or pork, feel free to continue doing so using these recipes. Take care to prepare meat in healthful ways, by broiling, grilling, roasting, or sautéing in extra virgin olive oil rather than in butter.

Beef Kebabs with Peanut Dipping Sauce

Remember when you were young, and you thought everything tasted better with a little peanut butter on it? Well, after tasting this recipe, you'll be sure you were absolutely right.

1/2 cup light soy sauce

2 tablespoons granulated brown sugar substitute (see note on page 326)

2 tablespoons sugar substitute

4 cloves garlic, pressed

1 1/2 pounds sirloin steak, 1 1/2" thick, cut into 1" pieces

1/2 cup creamy unsweetened natural peanut butter

3/4 cup water

3 tablespoons lime juice

1 tablespoon finely chopped ginger

1/4 teaspoon ground red pepper

1 green bell pepper, cut into squares

1 red bell pepper, cut into squares

1 large onion, cut into wedges

In a shallow dish, combine half of the soy sauce, 1 tablespoon of the brown sugar substitute, 1 tablespoon of the sugar substitute, and 2 of the pressed garlic cloves. Add the steak and stir to coat. Let stand for 20 minutes, stirring once.

Meanwhile, in a heavy saucepan over high heat, combine the peanut butter, water, lime juice, ginger,

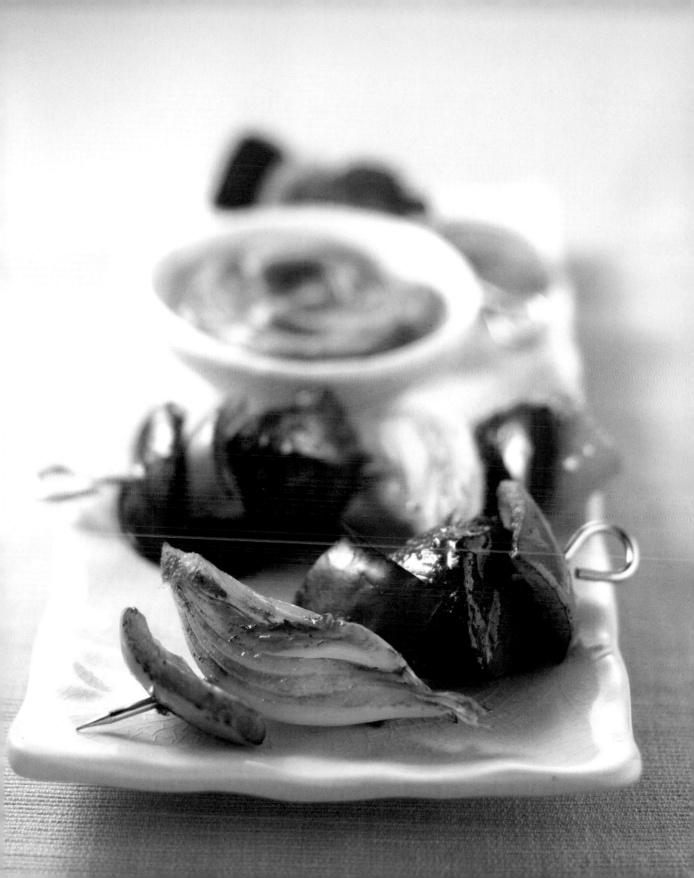

ground red pepper, the remaining half of the soy sauce, the remaining 1 tablespoon brown sugar substitute, the remaining 1 tablespoon sugar substitute, and the remaining 2 cloves pressed garlic. Cook, stirring constantly, until the mixture boils. Remove it from the heat.

Coat a grill rack with cooking spray. Preheat the grill to high.

Thread the steak, peppers, and onion onto four metal skewers. Place on the grill rack and cook, turning occasionally, for 10 minutes, or until the steak is no longer pink, and a thermometer inserted in the thickest portion registers 160°F and the juices run clear. Serve with the peanut sauce.

Makes 4 servings

NUTRITION AT A GLANCE

Per serving: 481 calories, 23 g fat, 6 g saturated fat, 46 g protein, 23 g carbohydrate, 4 g dietary fiber, 104 mg cholesterol, 863 mg sodium

THE BILTMORE HOTEL

1200 Anastasia Avenue, Coral Gables, Florida

EXECUTIVE CHEF GEOFFREY COUSINEAU

THE HISTORIC *BILTMORE HOTEL* IN CORAL GABLES IS A NATIONAL LANDMARK, THE ONLY RESORT IN SOUTH FLORIDA TO HAVE THAT DISTINCTIVE HONOR.

Grilled Lamb Loin Salad with Chilled Greek Olive Ratatouille

PHASE 1

Lamb

1 1/2 pounds lamb loin, trimmed of all visible fat

1 teaspoon extra virgin olive oil

2 tablespoons harissa paste

Kosher salt

Fresh black pepper

Ratatouille

1 zucchini, chopped

1 yellow squash, chopped

1   red bell pepper, chopped

1   yellow bell pepper, chopped

1   Japanese eggplant, chopped

1/2 bulb fennel, chopped

2   ounces chopped fresh garlic

1   teaspoon extra virgin olive oil

1   tablespoon tomato paste

Salt

Pepper

1   teaspoon chopped fresh rosemary

1   teaspoon chopped fresh basil

1   teaspoon chopped fresh oregano

2   ounces aged balsamic vinegar

2   ounces pitted Greek olives, chopped, for garnish

4   ounces crumbled feta cheese, for garnish

1   ounce basil-infused olive oil, for garnish

8   sprigs fennel, for garnish

To make the lamb: Rub the lamb with the olive oil, harissa paste, kosher salt and black pepper. Wrap with plastic wrap and refrigerate overnight.

To make the ratatouille: Sauté the zucchini, squash, peppers, eggplant, fennel, and garlic in the olive oil until soft but not overcooked. Drain off excess liquid and stir in tomato paste. Cook 1 more minute. Lightly season with salt and pepper. Add the rosemary, basil, oregano, and 1 ounce of the vinegar. Place in a glass or stainless steel bowl and refrigerate overnight.

To serve: Preheat the grill.

Grill the lamb to the desired temperature and let rest for 10 minutes before slicing. Firmly press the chilled ratatouille into a ring mold (or a nice round dollop in the center of the plate if no mold is available) with a spoon, dividing up into 8 plates. Slice the lamb and arrange on top of the ratatouille. Garnish with the olives, cheese, remaining balsamic vinegar, basil-infused olive oil, and fennel sprigs.

Makes 8 servings

NUTRITION AT A GLANCE

Per serving: 254 calories, 13 g fat, 4 g saturated fat, 23 g protein, 13 g carbohydrate, 3 g dietary fiber, 61 mg cholesterol, 349 mg sodium

Steak and Mushroom Kebabs

Whether you're planning to spend tomorrow by the pool or in the backyard, these tasty kebabs will fit in perfectly.

1/2	cup dry red wine
1/4	cup extra virgin olive oil
2	tablespoons South Beach Ketchup (see page 242)
1	tablespoon vinegar
1	teaspoon Worcestershire sauce
1	clove garlic
1	teaspoon salt
1/2	teaspoon dried marjoram
1/2	teaspoon dried oregano
2	pounds sirloin steak, cut into 2" pieces
2	cups large mushrooms

In a large bowl, combine the wine, oil, ketchup, vinegar, Worcestershire sauce, garlic, salt, marjoram, and oregano. Add the steak and the mushrooms and stir to coat. Cover and allow to stand at room temperature for 20 minutes, then refrigerate overnight.

Coat a grill rack or broiler-pan rack with cooking spray. Preheat the grill or broiler.

Drain and discard the marinade. Thread the meat and the mushrooms onto 4 metal skewers.

Grill over hot coals or broil 4" from the heat, turning occasionally, for 7 minutes, or until the meat is no longer pink.

Makes 4 servings

NUTRITION AT A GLANCE

Per serving: 350 calories, 11 g fat, 5 g saturated fat, 50 g protein, 5 g carbohydrate, 1 g dietary fiber, 138 mg cholesterol, 819 mg sodium

Beef Fondue

If you have time, try making an assortment of the South Beach sauces in this book, then serving them as accompaniments to this wonderfully flavorful fondue for beef tenderloin. It's the perfect fare for company.

2 pounds beef tenderloin, cut into 1" cubes

1 recipe South Beach Teriyaki Sauce (see page 241)

1 recipe South Beach Tomato Sauce (see page 234)

1 recipe South Beach Barbecue Sauce (see page 239)

1 recipe South Beach Cocktail Sauce (see page 240)

1 recipe South Beach Ketchup (see page 242)

Canola oil or beef or chicken broth

Evenly divide the beef among 4 individual dishes. Place the sauces in individual bowls. Heat the oil or broth in a fondue pot to about 375°F. Using skewers, dip the beef tenderloin cubes into the hot oil or broth to cook it. Then dip the beef into one of the sauces.

Makes 4 servings

NUTRITION AT A GLANCE

Per serving: 348 calories, 16 g fat, 6 g saturated fat, 47 g protein, 0 g carbohydrate, 0 g dietary fiber, 142 mg cholesterol, 106 mg sodium

Filet Mignon with Tomato Topping

You can enjoy this tender cut of beef in all phases of the South Beach Diet. Here, it's served topped with juicy tomatoes gently marinated in a mixture of garlic, herbs, and soy.

2	teaspoons light soy sauce
1 1/2	teaspoons Dijon mustard
1 1/2	teaspoons finely chopped parsley
1	clove garlic, minced
2	tomatoes, finely chopped
2	teaspoons extra virgin olive oil
4	steaks filet mignon (6 ounces each and 1 1/2 " thick)
1/4	teaspoon salt
1/2	teaspoon ground black pepper

Preheat the oven to 400°F.

In a bowl, combine the soy sauce, mustard, parsley, and garlic. Gently stir in the tomatoes.

Heat the oil in a large ovenproof heavy skillet over high heat. Season the steaks with the salt and pepper. Place the steaks in the pan and cook on one side for 4 minutes, or until deeply browned. Turn and brown the second side for 30 seconds. Place the skillet in the oven and cook for 12 minutes, or until a thermometer inserted in the thickest portion registers 160°F for medium. Serve topped with the tomatoes.

Makes 4 servings

NUTRITION AT A GLANCE

Per serving: 304 calories, 16 g fat, 5 g saturated fat, 36 g protein, 2 g carbohydrate, 0 g dietary fiber, 105 mg cholesterol, 389 mg sodium

Marinated Steak

Lean meats don't have to be boring. You can stir-fry vegetables to go with this entrée. Put these steaks in the refrigerator before going to work, and you can prepare your meal in 15 minutes when you get home.

- 1/2 cup dry red wine
- 2 teaspoons light soy sauce
- Pinch of ground black pepper
- 1/4 teaspoon dried oregano
- 1 pound flank steak, trimmed of all visible fat

In a shallow dish, combine the wine, soy sauce, pepper, and oregano. Add the steak and turn to coat both sides with the marinade. Cover and refrigerate overnight, turning the steak occasionally.

When ready to cook, remove the steak from the marinade, pat dry with paper towels, and discard the marinade.

Coat a broiler-pan rack with olive oil cooking spray. Preheat the broiler.

Place the steaks on the prepared rack. Broil 4" from the heat source for 5 minutes per side, or until a thermometer inserted in the center of the steak registers 160°F for medium.

To serve, thinly slice the steak diagonally across the grain and place on a serving plate.

Makes 4 servings

NUTRITION AT A GLANCE

Per serving: 179 calories, 8 g fat, 4 g saturated fat, 22 g protein, 0 g carbohydrate, 0 g dietary fiber, 54 mg cholesterol, 118 mg sodium

Steak au Poivre

This is our South Beach version of a favorite recipe.

> 1 clove garlic, crushed
>
> 1 1/2 teaspoons crushed black or mixed peppercorns
>
> 4 beef tenderloin steaks (4 ounces each), trimmed of all visible fat
>
> 1/4 onion, chopped
>
> 2/3 cup green bell pepper strips
>
> 2/3 cup red bell pepper strips
>
> 2/3 cup yellow bell pepper strips
>
> 1 clove garlic, minced
>
> 1/2 teaspoon beef-flavored bouillon granules
>
> 1/2 teaspoon ground paprika
>
> 1/3 cup water
>
> 1/3 cup fat-free evaporated milk

In a small bowl, combine the crushed garlic and 1 teaspoon of the peppercorns. Press a small amount of the mixture onto each side of the steaks.

Heat a large nonstick skillet coated with olive oil cooking spray over medium heat. Arrange the steaks in the skillet so that they do not overlap. Cook the steaks, turning frequently, for 10 minutes, or until a thermometer inserted in the center of a steak registers 160°F for medium. Remove the steaks to a serving platter and keep warm.

Clean the skillet, coat with cooking spray, and place over medium heat. Add the onion, bell peppers, and minced garlic and cook, stirring occasionally, for 5 minutes. Spoon the mixture over the steaks.

In a small bowl, combine the bouillon granules, paprika, water, milk and the remaining 1/2 teaspoon peppercorns. Pour into the skillet and cook, stirring often, over medium heat until the mixture is reduced to 1/2 cup.

Spoon the sauce over each steak and serve immediately.

Makes 4 servings

NUTRITION AT A GLANCE
Per serving: 204 calories, 7 g fat, 3 g saturated fat, 21 g protein, 8 g carbohydrate, 1 g dietary fiber, 59 mg cholesterol, 72 mg sodium

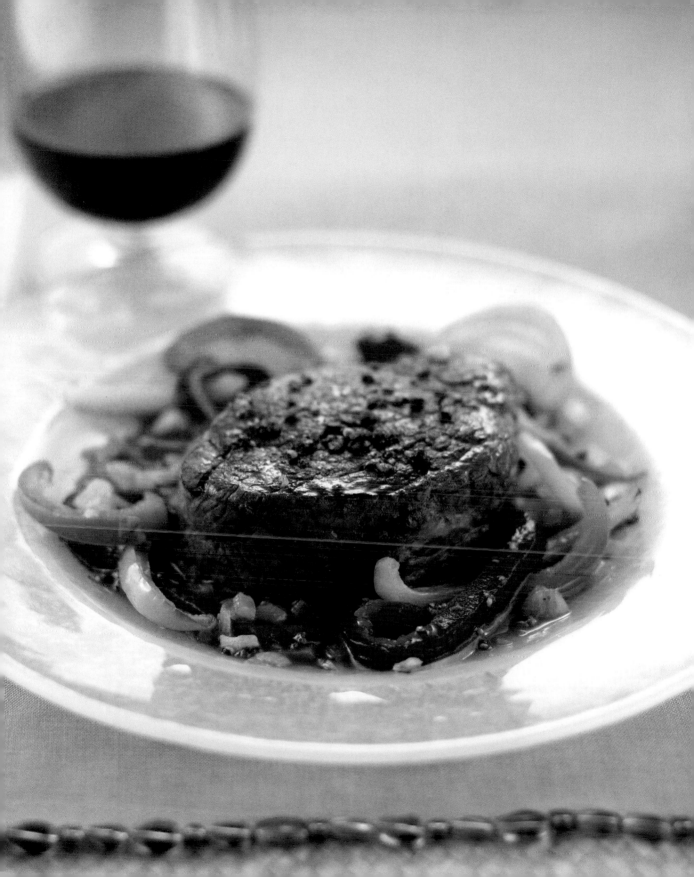

Sicilian Chopped Sirloin Steak

This lunch is a new twist on a plain old hamburger. In Phase 2, you can even add the whole wheat bun.

1 small head garlic

6 oil-packed sun-dried tomato halves, drained and finely chopped

2 tablespoons mayonnaise

1 1/2 pounds sirloin steak, trimmed of all visible fat, chopped

4 slices fontina cheese

Arugula, for garnish

Fresh basil leaves, for garnish

4 whole wheat buns (Phase 2 or 3)

Preheat the oven to 400°F.

Wrap the garlic in foil and roast for 30 minutes, or until very tender. When cool enough to handle, squeeze the garlic pulp into a cup. Add the sun-dried-tomato halves and mayonnaise. Add the steak and mix well.

Evenly divide the steak mixture into 4 equal parts and form into patties.

Heat a large nonstick skillet over medium heat. Add the patties and cook, turning occasionally, for 10 minutes, or until a thermometer inserted in the center registers 160°F and the meat is no longer pink. When the patties have been turned over for the last time, place a cheese slice onto each patty. When the cheese melts, remove the patties to 4 serving plates and garnish with the arugula and basil.

Makes 4 servings

NUTRITION AT A GLANCE

Per serving: 402 calories, 22 g fat, 9 g saturated fat, 44 g protein, 4 g carbohydrate, 0 g dietary fiber, 139 mg cholesterol, 376 mg sodium

Steak Diane

You will be "the shining star of the meal" when you serve this simple version of the classic tenderloin steak.

4	center-cut beef tenderloin medallions (3 ounces each), trimmed of all visible fat
	Salt
	Coarsely ground black pepper
1/4	cup + 1 tablespoon trans-free margarine
1/4	cup finely chopped shallots
1/4	cup mushroom caps, sliced 1/8" thick
1/8	teaspoon minced garlic
1	teaspoon mustard powder
1	tablespoon Worcestershire sauce
2	tablespoons lemon juice
2	tablespoons chopped parsley
1	tablespoon fresh chives

Place each steak, one at a time, between 2 pieces of waxed paper. Starting in the center and working your way to the outside, pound the steaks with a meat mallet until 1/2" thick. Dry the steaks with paper towels, then sprinkle with the salt and pepper.

In a large chafing dish over medium heat, melt 3 tablespoons of the margarine. Increase the heat to medium-high and cook each steak for 2 minutes on each side. Remove to a plate.

Melt the remaining 2 tablespoons margarine. Add the shallots, mushroom caps, and garlic and cook, stirring, for 1 minute. Add the mustard and Worcestershire sauce and mix well. Return the steaks to the pan, and cook until desired doneness. Place the steaks on warm serving plates. Add the lemon juice, parsley, and chives to the pan and mix thoroughly. Cook for 30 seconds, or until just warm. Pour the sauce evenly over the steaks.

Makes 4 servings

NUTRITION AT A GLANCE

Per serving: 397 calories, 21 g fat, 5 g saturated fat, 32 g protein, 28 g carbohydrate, 7 g dietary fiber, 43 mg cholesterol, 266 mg sodium

Pepper-Spiked Beef Stew

Braised beef spiked with red pepper, chili, and other seasonings makes this stew special. It freezes well, so you might want to simmer up a double batch. You can try substituting sweet potatoes or even butternut squash for the potatoes and carrots. Or, if you eliminate the potatoes, this recipe will fit into Phase 2.

- 2 tablespoons whole wheat flour
- 1 tablespoon chili powder
- 1/2 teaspoon salt
- 2 pounds lean round steak, top or bottom, trimmed of all visible fat and cubed
- 1 tablespoon extra virgin olive oil
- 3 onions, sliced
- 3 cloves garlic, minced
- 1 teaspoon dried oregano
- 2 cups beef broth
- 2 cans (14 1/2 ounces each) stewed tomatoes
- 1/2 teaspoon crushed red-pepper flakes
- 1 potato, scrubbed and cubed
- 4 carrots, sliced

In a large zip-top plastic bag, combine the flour, 1 teaspoon of the chili powder, and the salt. Add the beef, seal the bag, and toss to coat well.

Heat the oil in a large saucepan over medium-high heat. Add the beef and cook, stirring occasionally, for 7 minutes, or until browned. Add the onions, garlic, and oregano. Reduce the heat to medium and cook, stirring often, for 5 minutes.

Add the broth, tomatoes (with juice), red-pepper flakes, and the remaining 2 teaspoons chili powder. Bring to a boil. Reduce the heat to low, cover, and simmer for 2 hours, stirring occasionally, or until the beef is almost tender.

Add the potato and carrots. Cover and cook for 30 minutes, or until the vegetables are tender.

Makes 8 servings

NUTRITION AT A GLANCE

Per serving: 190 calories, 5 g fat, 1 1/2 g saturated fat, 24 g protein, 19 g carbohydrate, 4 g dietary fiber, 45 mg cholesterol, 440 mg sodium

Roasted Eggplant Stuffed with Beef

The presentation for this dish looks elaborate, but its preparation is really quite easy. You can prepare the stuffing mixture ahead and fill the eggplant shells just before roasting.

2	eggplants (16 ounces each)
2	tablespoons extra virgin olive oil
1/2	large onion, chopped
1	green bell pepper, chopped
2	cloves garlic, minced
1	pound extra-lean ground beef
1 1/2	teaspoons dried oregano
1/2	cup tomato sauce
1/2	cup (2 ounces) grated Parmesan cheese
1/4	teaspoon salt
1/4	teaspoon ground black pepper

Preheat the oven to 400°F.

Pierce the eggplants in 2 or 3 places and place on a baking sheet. Roast, turning once or twice, for 20 minutes, or just until tender. When cool enough to handle, halve lengthwise and scoop out the pulp, leaving a 1/2" to 3/4" shell. Set the shells aside. Chop the pulp and let drain in a colander in the sink.

Heat 1 tablespoon of the oil in a large skillet over medium heat. Add the onion and bell pepper and cook, stirring occasionally, for 8 minutes, or until tender. Add the garlic and beef and cook, stirring to crumble the beef, for 5 minutes, or until no longer pink. Stir in the eggplant pulp, oregano, and tomato sauce. Reduce the heat to low and cook, stirring occasionally, for 15 minutes, or until thick. Stir in 1/4 cup of the cheese, the salt, and black pepper.

Place the eggplant shells on a baking sheet and evenly divide the beef mixture among them. Sprinkle with the remaining 1/4 cup cheese and drizzle with the remaining 1 tablespoon oil. Roast for 15 minutes, or until lightly browned on top.

Makes 4 servings

NUTRITION AT A GLANCE

Per serving: 342 calories, 17 g fat, 6 g saturated fat, 31 g protein, 21 g carbohydrate, 7 g dietary fiber, 71 mg cholesterol, 677 mg sodium

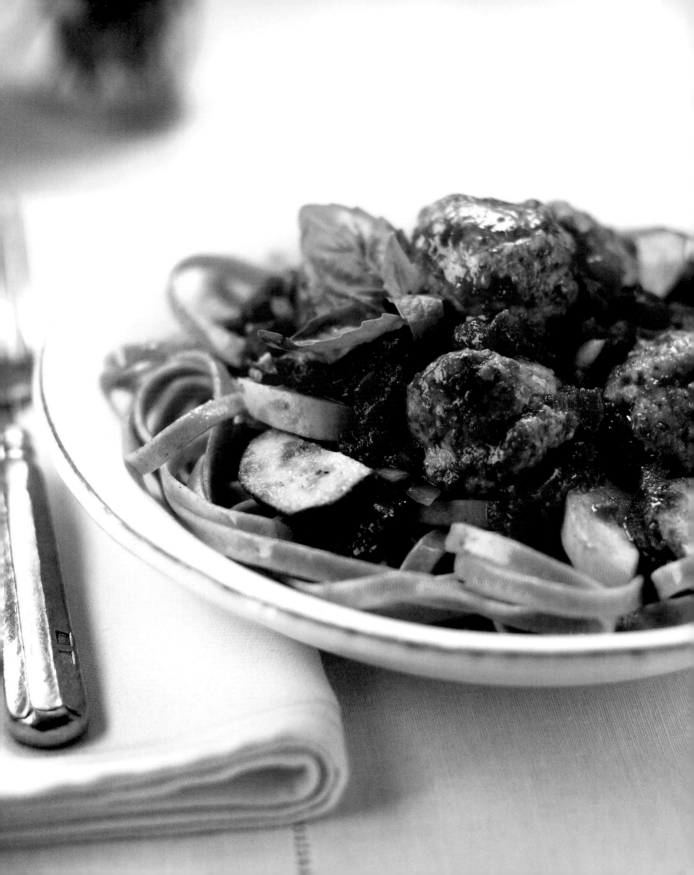

Meatballs with Tomato and Zucchini Medley

Use this one-dish meal to easily add a few servings of vegetables to your day. Serve it in bowls with crusty whole grain bread or spoon it over whole wheat fettuccine.

1/2	pound extra-lean ground beef or ground turkey breast
1/4	cup whole wheat bread crumbs
1/4	cup liquid egg substitute or 1 egg
3/4	teaspoon ground black pepper
1/2	teaspoon dried Italian seasoning
6	tablespoons grated Parmesan cheese
1	onion, finely chopped
2	cloves garlic, minced
2	zucchini, halved lengthwise and sliced
1	yellow squash, halved lengthwise and sliced
1	can (16 ounces) Italian-style cut tomatoes
1	can (16 ounces) crushed tomatoes
1/4	cup chopped fresh basil
	Sprig basil, for garnish

In a large bowl, combine the beef or turkey, bread crumbs, egg substitute or egg, 1/2 teaspoon of the pepper, the Italian seasoning, and 4 tablespoons of the cheese. Form into balls the size of walnuts.

Spray a large nonstick skillet with cooking spray and heat over medium heat. Working in batches, add the meatballs and cook for 15 minutes, or until browned and no longer pink inside. Remove to a bowl, leaving drippings in the skillet. Repeat to cook the remaining meatballs.

In the same skillet in warm drippings over medium-high heat, add the onion and garlic and cook for 5 minutes, or until the onion is tender. Stir in the zucchini, yellow squash, cut tomatoes (with juice), crushed tomatoes, the remaining 1/4 teaspoon pepper, the remaining 2 tablespoons cheese, and the meatballs. Heat to boiling. Reduce the heat to low, cover, and cook for 20 minutes. Stir in the chopped basil. Garnish with the basil sprig.

Makes 4 servings

NUTRITION AT A GLANCE

Per serving: 280 calories, 20 g fat, 5 g saturated fat, 23 g protein, 25 g carbohydrate, 6 g dietary fiber, 88 mg cholesterol, 646 mg sodium

New Beef Burgundy

This version of the familiar French boeuf bourguignonne is simple yet sophisticated. Beef, burgundy, onions, and mushrooms are the hallmarks of this favorite dish. For a twist, there's even a surprise ingredient: unsweetened cocoa powder!

1/4	cup whole wheat flour
1/4	teaspoon salt
1/4	teaspoon ground black pepper
1 1/2	pounds round steak, top or bottom, cubed
2	tablespoons extra virgin olive oil
1/2	pound pearl onions
1	pound mushrooms, quartered
3	cloves garlic, minced
3	cups burgundy wine
4	cups beef broth
1/4	cup tomato paste
1	teaspoon unsweetened cocoa powder
2	bay leaves
1/4	cup Italian parsley, chopped

In a zip-top plastic bag, combine the flour, salt, and pepper. Add the beef, seal the bag, and toss to coat well.

Heat 1 tablespoon of the oil in a large saucepan over medium-high heat. Working in batches to prevent overcrowding the pan, add the beef and cook, stirring frequently, for 5 minutes, or until browned. Remove to a plate and repeat with remaining beef.

Add the remaining 1 tablespoon oil to the pan. Add the onions, mushrooms, and garlic and cook, stirring often, for 10 minutes, or until lightly browned.

Add the wine, broth, tomato paste, cocoa powder, bay leaves, and beef. Bring to a boil. Reduce the heat to low, cover, and simmer for 2 hours. Remove and discard the bay leaves. Sprinkle with the parsley.

Makes 8 servings

NUTRITION AT A GLANCE
Per serving: 270 calories, 10 g fat, 3 g saturated fat, 20 g protein, 11 g carbohydrate, 2 g dietary fiber, 45 mg cholesterol, 690 mg sodium

South Beach Meat Loaf with Vegetables

Brown rice helps keeps this meat loaf moist and lends a pleasing nutty flavor that you won't find in traditional versions.

1	tablespoon extra virgin olive oil or vegetable oil
1	onion, chopped
1/2	red bell pepper, chopped
1/2	green bell pepper, chopped
1/2	pound extra-lean ground beef
1/2	pound ground turkey breast
1	cup chunky salsa
1	egg, beaten
3/4	teaspoon salt
1/2	teaspoon ground black pepper
1	clove garlic, minced
1/2	cup cooked brown rice

Preheat the oven to 350°F.

Heat the oil in a small skillet over medium heat. Add the onion and bell peppers and cook for 5 minutes, or until tender.

In a large bowl, combine the beef, turkey, salsa, egg, salt, black pepper, and garlic. Stir in the vegetables and rice. Place the mixture in a round baking dish and pat into an oblong loaf.

Bake for 45 minutes, or until a thermometer inserted in the center registers 160°F and the meat is no longer pink.

Makes 6 servings

NUTRITION AT A GLANCE

Per serving: 225 calories, 10 g fat, 3 g saturated fat, 17 g protein, 16 g carbohydrate, 1 g dietary fiber, 79 mg cholesterol, 366 mg sodium

From the Menu of . . .
SMITH & WOLLENSKY
1 Washington Avenue, Miami Beach

CHEF ROBERT MIGNOLA

SMITH & WOLLENSKY IS ON THE SOUTHERN TIP OF MIAMI BEACH, FACING FISHER ISLAND AND LOOKING OUT OVER THE BAY. THE VIEWS ARE SPECTACULAR.

Grilled Filet Mignon with Roasted Garlic and Chipotle Pepper Chimichurri
PHASE 1

Filet Mignon

4 filet mignons (6 ounces each)

Salt

Fresh ground black pepper

Roasted Garlic and Chipotle Pepper Chimichurri (recipe next page)

Roasted Garlic and Chipotle Pepper Chimichurri

1	head garlic
1	chipotle pepper in adobo sauce
1/4	cup extra virgin olive oil
1/4	cup finely chopped flat-leaf parsley
	Salt
	Fresh ground black pepper

To make the filet mignon: Preheat the grill.

Season the steaks with salt and pepper. Grill the steaks to desired doneness, about 4 to 6 minutes per side for medium-rare. Drizzle with chimichurri sauce. Chimichurri goes great with any grilled beef, pork, chicken, or even fish dish.

To make the chimichurri: Preheat the oven to 325°F.

Cut the top 1/4 " off the garlic to expose the cloves, wrap loosely in aluminum foil, and bake for approximately 45 minutes until the garlic is lightly browned and very soft. Cool to room temperature, then squeeze out the roasted garlic.

Combine the garlic with the chipotle pepper in a food processor or blender, slowly drizzle in the oil, then stir in the parsley and season with salt and pepper.

Note: Chipotle peppers are very spicy. Use more or less according to taste.

Makes 4 servings

NUTRITION AT A GLANCE

Per serving: 420 calories, 25 g fat, 6 g saturated fat, 39 g protein, 7 g carbohydrate, 0 g dietary fiber, 115 mg cholesterol, 390 mg sodium

Pizza Meat Pie

Everyone has heard of pizza that's amoré. *After all, what's not to love about this recipe?*

1	pound extra-lean ground beef
1/2	cup non-fat dry milk
1/2	cup whole wheat bread crumbs
1	teaspoon salt
1/2	teaspoon ground black pepper
1	clove garlic, crushed
1	cup (4 ounces) shredded reduced-fat mozzarella cheese
2	tablespoons tomato paste
1/2	cup water
1	can (4 ounces) sliced mushrooms, undrained
1	teaspoon dried oregano
2	tablespoons finely chopped onion
1/3	cup (1 1/2 ounces) grated Parmesan cheese

Preheat the oven to 350°F.

In a medium bowl, combine the beef, milk, bread crumbs, salt, pepper, and garlic. Mix well. Pat the mixture into a 9" pie plate.

In the same bowl, combine the mozzarella cheese, tomato paste, water, mushrooms (with juice), oregano, and onion; mix well. Spoon the mixture over the meat mixture in the pan. Sprinkle with the Parmesan cheese.

Bake for 35 to 40 minutes, or until the meat is no longer pink.

Makes 4 servings

NUTRITION AT A GLANCE

Per serving: 382 calories, 18 g fat, 8 g saturated fat, 38 g protein, 17 g carbohydrate, 2 g dietary fiber, 61 mg cholesterol, 1,221 mg sodium

Mexican Lasagna

Try this lasagna when you're in the mood for Mexican.

1	pound extra lean ground beef or turkey breast
1/2	large onion, chopped
1	large clove garlic, minced
1 1/2	cups low-fat cottage cheese
1	cup fat-free sour cream
1	jar (4 ounces) chopped green chile peppers
1/2	cup chopped cilantro (optional)
2	teaspoons ground cumin
1/8	teaspoon salt
2 1/2	cups salsa
4	whole wheat tortillas (6" in diameter), halved
1 1/4	cup (5 ounces) shredded, reduced-fat Monterey Jack cheeses

Preheat the oven to 350°F.

Coat a 13" × 9" baking dish with cooking spray.

Coat a large nonstick skillet with cooking spray, and place over medium heat. Add the ground beef or turkey and cook, turning several times, for 5 minutes or until no longer pink.

Remove the ground beef or turkey to a medium bowl. Wipe the skillet with a paper towel. Coat the skillet with cooking spray. Place over medium heat. Add the onion and garlic. Cover and cook, stirring occasionally, for 7 to 8 minutes, or until lightly browned. Add to the ground beef or turkey in the bowl.

In another medium bowl, combine the cottage cheese, sour cream, peppers, cilantro (if using), cumin, and salt.

Spread 1 cup of the salsa across the bottom of the baking dish. Arrange half of the tortillas evenly over the salsa. Spread half of the cheese over the tortillas. Top with half of the ground beef or turkey mixture. Top with 1 cup of the remaining salsa and 1/2 cup of the Monterey Jack cheese. Repeat the layering sequence with the remaining tortillas, cheese, and ground beef or turkey mixture. Sprinkle with the remaining salsa and 3/4 cup Monterey Jack cheese.

Bake for 30 minutes, or until heated through. Loosely cover with foil if the cheese browns too quickly.

Makes 8 servings

NUTRITION AT A GLANCE

Per serving: 250 calories, 8 g fat, 4 g saturated fat, 24 g protein, 24 g carbohydrate, 3 g dietary fiber, 50 mg cholesterol, 840 mg sodium

NORMAN'S

21 Almeria Avenue, Coral Gables, Florida

CHEF NORMAN VAN AKEN

THE MENU AT *NORMAN'S* FEATURES DISHES WITH
AN INVENTIVE MIX OF FLAVORS—A BLEND OF LATIN,
NORTH AMERICAN, CARIBBEAN, AND ASIAN—KNOWN
AS NEW WORLD CUISINE. THESE TASTY PORK CHOPS
ARE A PERFECT EXAMPLE.

Bolivian Spiced Pork Chops

PHASE 1

Split Peas

2 1/2	tablespoons extra virgin olive oil
2	cloves garlic, minced
1/2	onion, finely chopped
2	ribs celery, finely chopped
1	carrot, finely chopped
1	teaspoon ground red pepper
1	teaspoon ground cumin
4	cups chicken broth

1	smoked ham hock
1	bay leaf, broken in half
1	package (12 ounces) split peas

Pork Chops

1 1/2	tablespoons ground cumin
3	teaspoons ground cardamom
3	teaspoons ground coriander
1/2	tablespoon ground red pepper
3	tablespoons lemon peel
1/2	tablespoon kosher salt
1/2	tablespoon pepper
6	loin pork chops, 1 1/2" thick
3	tablespoons roasted garlic oil or extra virgin olive oil

To make the peas: In a medium saucepan over medium-low heat, add the olive oil. When hot, add the garlic and cook for 30 seconds. Turn up the heat to medium-high and add the onion, celery, and carrot. When they start to turn golden, add the red pepper and cumin. Stir and add the chicken broth, ham, bay leaf, and peas. Bring to a simmer, turn down the heat, and cook until the peas are cooked, about 45 minutes. Remove the bay leaf and discard.

Mash the split pea mixture. This will thicken as it cools.

To make the pork: Preheat the oven to 350°F.

In a small bowl, combine the cumin, cardamom, coriander, red pepper, lemon peel, salt, and pepper. Place the pork chops in a zip-top plastic bag. Sprinkle the spice mixture over the pork chops and rub it on both sides.

Heat a skillet to medium-high heat. Add the oil and sear the chops on both sides. As they brown, put them on a half-sheet pan and finish them in the oven to the desired doneness.

Note: I like to garnish this with sliced stuffed green olives and lemon wedges.

Makes 6 servings

NUTRITION AT A GLANCE

Per serving: 453 calories, 20 g fat, 4 g saturated fat, 28 g protein, 42 g carbohydrate, 11 g dietary fiber, 36 mg cholesterol, 800 mg sodium

Sage and Rosemary Pork

Butterflying the pork loin open, filling it, and then rolling it back up is a great way to infuse flavor into the loin. This recipe is perfect when you're having guests for dinner.

Filling

2	tablespoons chopped parsley
1 1/2	tablespoons chopped fresh sage or thyme leaves
1	tablespoon chopped fresh rosemary
3	cloves garlic, minced
3	tablespoons extra virgin olive oil
2	teaspoons Dijon mustard
1/4	teaspoon salt
1/4	teaspoon ground black pepper

Pork Loin

1	boneless center loin pork roast (about 2 pounds)
3/4	teaspoon salt
1/2	teaspoon ground black pepper
1	tablespoon extra virgin olive oil
	Fresh sage leaves, for garnish
	Sprigs rosemary, for garnish

To make the filling: In a small bowl, combine the parsley, sage or thyme, rosemary, garlic, oil, mustard, salt, and pepper.

To make the pork loin: Preheat the oven to 350°F.

Butterfly the pork loin. Sprinkle the top side of the butterflied loin with half of the salt and pepper. Spread the filling evenly across the loin, leaving a 1/2" border along the edge where you made the first cut.

Beginning at the opposite edge, roll the loin up to wrap the filling. Using kitchen twine, tie the loin every 1 1/2" to hold its shape.

Rub the loin with the oil and sprinkle with the remaining salt and pepper. Place the loin in a small roasting pan and position on the center rack of the oven. Roast for 1 hour, or until a thermometer inserted in the center registers 155°F and the juices run clear. Let stand for 10 minutes before carving. To prevent slices from unrolling, skewer the roast every 1/4" with wooden picks along the edge where the roll ends. Slice crosswise between the wooden picks and ties. Remove the kitchen twine before serving. Garnish with the sage leaves and rosemary sprigs.

Makes 6 servings

NUTRITION AT A GLANCE

Per serving: 306 calories, 19 g fat, 5 g saturated fat, 31 g protein, 1 g carbohydrate, 0 g dietary fiber, 97 mg cholesterol, 506 mg sodium

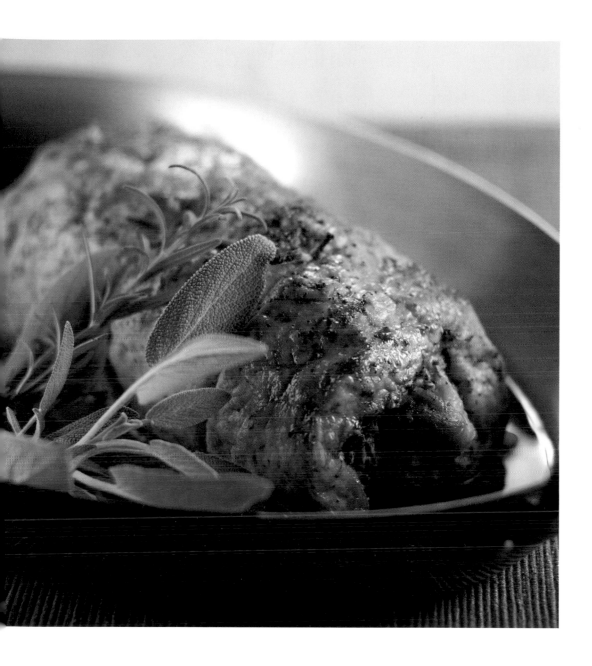

Garlic and Soy Grilled Pork Chops

Grill up chunks of fresh vegetables alongside these lip-smacking pork chops for an irresistible outdoor feast. Bell pepper, sweet onion, and zucchini would work quite nicely.

4 boneless center-cut pork loin chops, trimmed of all visible fat
1 tablespoon light soy sauce
2 teaspoons minced garlic
1/2 teaspoon paprika
1/2 teaspoon salt
1/4 teaspoon ground black pepper
Fresh herbs, for garnish

Sprinkle the pork chops all over with soy sauce, garlic, paprika, salt, and pepper. Cover and refrigerate at least 20 minutes or up to 2 hours.

Coat a grill rack or broiler-pan rack with cooking spray. Preheat the grill or broiler.

Cook the pork chops 4" from the heat, turning once halfway through cooking time, for 10 to 12 minutes, or until a thermometer inserted in the center of a chop registers 155°F and the juices run clear. Garnish with the herbs.

Makes 4 servings

NUTRITION AT A GLANCE

Per serving: 70 calories, 2 g fat, 0 g saturated fat, 11 g protein, 1 g carbohydrate, 0 g dietary fiber, 30 mg cholesterol, 436 mg sodium

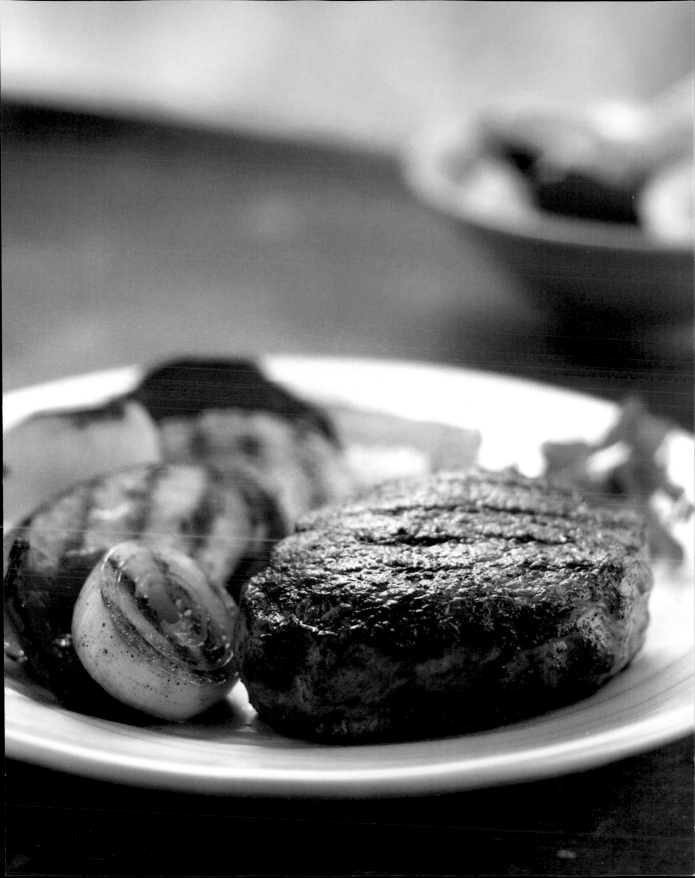

From the Menu of . . .
TIMO
17624 Collins Avenue, Sunny Isles, Florida

EXECUTIVE CHEF TIM ANDRIOLA

TIMO IS A HANDSOME BISTRO CO-OWNED BY ACCLAIMED CHEF TIM ANDRIOLA. ITALIAN FOR THYME, *TIMO'S* MENU SPOTLIGHTS ANDRIOLA'S FLAIR AND APPRECIATION FOR THE FLAVORS OF ITALY AND THE MEDITERRANEAN.

Roasted Pork Tenderloin with Chickpeas, Roasted Peppers, and Clams
PHASE 2

1/2	cup orange juice
1	tablespoon lime juice
1/4	cup + 2 tablespoons vegetable oil
2	tablespoons whole grain mustard
1	tablespoon chopped garlic
1/2	tablespoon paprika
1	tablespoon chopped fresh thyme leaves
1/2	tablespoon black peppercorns

1   whole pork tenderloin (about 3/4–1 pound), silver
    skin removed and trimmed of all visible fat

Salt

Pepper

1   tablespoon minced shallot

1   bulb garlic (about 10–12 cloves)

1/4   cup roasted red and yellow peppers (skin and seeds
      removed), diced

2   tablespoons tomato concassé (peeled, cooked
    tomatoes)

1   cup cooked chickpeas

3/4   cup chicken broth

12   littleneck clams

1   tablespoon chopped parsley

In a large bowl, combine the orange juice, lime juice, 1/4 cup vegetable oil, mustard, chopped garlic, paprika, thyme, and peppercorns. Submerge the pork in this marinade for a minimum of 6 to 8 hours, preferably overnight. Remove the pork from the marinade and pat dry with paper towels. Season with the salt and pepper.

Preheat the oven to 350°F.

Heat the 2 tablespoons vegetable oil in an ovenproof heavy sauté pan on medium-high heat. Sauté the shallot and bulb of garlic for 3 to 5 minutes, until lightly browned. Add the pork, brown evenly and then place in the oven for 10 to 15 minutes.

Remove the pan from the oven. Remove the pork from the pan and place in a warm spot to rest for a few minutes. In the same sauté pan on medium heat, add the peppers, tomato, chickpeas, and broth and bring to a simmer. Add the clams and cover tightly. When the clams open, remove them to serving plates. Add the parsley to the sauté pan and adjust seasoning with salt and pepper. Spoon the chickpea mixture into the center of the plates. Slice the pork into 1/4 " slices and arrange them on top of the chickpeas.

Makes 4 servings

NUTRITION AT A GLANCE

Per serving: 492 calories, 27 g fat, 3 g saturated fat, 35 g protein, 29 g carbohydrate, 5 g dietary fiber, 87 mg cholesterol, 543 mg sodium

Sesame Pork Tenderloin

The sesame seeds provide a unique mild, nutty flavor to the pork tenderloin.

             2 lean pork tenderloins (about 3/4–1 pound each)
         1/4 cup extra virgin olive oil
         1/4 cup sesame seeds
             1 rib celery, chopped
             2 tablespoons chopped onion
             1 cup whole wheat bread crumbs
             1 teaspoon lemon juice
             1 teaspoon Worcestershire sauce
         1/2 teaspoon salt
         1/2 teaspoon dried thyme
         1/8 teaspoon ground black pepper

Preheat the oven to 325°F.

Cut each tenderloin almost through lengthwise, then flatten.

Heat the oil in a large skillet over medium-high heat. Add the sesame seeds, celery, and onion and cook, stirring frequently, for 3 minutes, or until lightly browned. Add the bread crumbs, lemon juice, Worcestershire sauce, salt, thyme, and pepper. Toss lightly. Spread the stuffing on the cut surface of 1 tenderloin. Place the second tenderloin, cut side down on top of the stuffing. Fasten the tenderloins together with kitchen string or skewers. Place in an open roasting pan.

Roast for 1 hour and 20 minutes, or until a thermometer inserted in the center registers 155°F and the juices run clear. Let stand for 10 minutes before slicing.

Makes 6 servings

NUTRITION AT A GLANCE

Per serving: 377 calories, 18 g fat, 3 g saturated fat, 35 g protein, 15 g carbohydrate, 0 g dietary fiber, 114 mg cholesterol, 442 mg sodium

From the Menu of . . .

BLUE DOOR
AT DELANO

1685 Collins Avenue, Miami Beach

CHEF CLAUDE TROISGROS

Located in the Delano Hotel, one of
Miami Beach's hip hotels, *Blue Door at Delano*
was named one of America's best new restaurants
for 1998 by *Esquire* magazine. In a chic, art deco
setting, consulting chef Claude Troisgros
has teamed with Chef Damon Gordon
to produce modern, French–based cuisine
with a tropical influence.

Veal Mignon
PHASE 3

8   baby artichokes

1/3   cup chopped shallots

1/3   cup chopped garlic

1/3   cup extra virgin olive oil

1/4   cup soy sauce

12   medallions of veal (2 1/2 ounces each)

1/2   cup sun-dried tomatoes, julienned

1/3   cup capers

1/3   cup raisins

Chopped parsley

Salt

Pepper

Fresh thyme (optional)

In a saucepan, cook the artichokes in water until tender, about 20 minutes. Allow the artichokes to cool and then remove the top and outer leaves and cut them into quarters.

In a sauté pan, lightly sauté the shallots and garlic in 3 tablespoons of the olive oil until tender. Add the soy sauce and slightly reduce. Remove the sauce from the pan and set aside.

In the sauté pan, sauté the veal in the remaining olive oil until medium-rare. Remove to a warm platter. Sauté the artichokes, tomatoes, capers, and raisins in olive oil and season with the parsley, salt, and pepper to taste.

Place 3 pieces of veal on each plate, divide the artichoke mixture on top, and spoon the sauce over the top.

Garnish with the thyme, if using.

Makes 4 servings

NUTRITION AT A GLANCE

Per serving: 365 calories, 22 g fat, 3 g saturated fat, 17 g protein, 32 g carbohydrate, 12 g dietary fiber, 32 mg cholesterol, 909 mg sodium

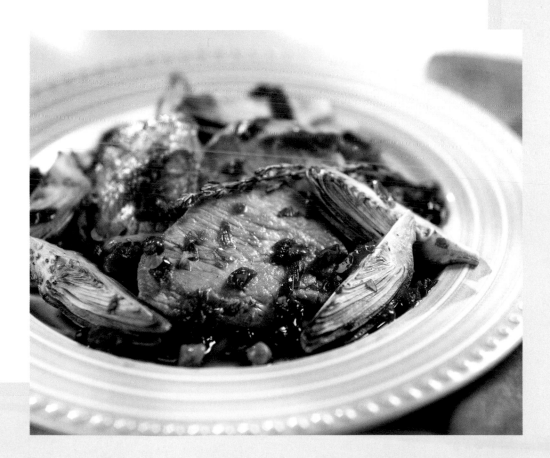

MY SOUTH BEACH DIET

FOR THE FIRST TIME, I TRULY UNDERSTAND "EAT TO LIVE, NOT LIVE TO EAT."

I reached my highest weight ever last year at 248 pounds. On top of that, I was taking medication for high blood pressure, arthritis, and anxiety, as well as a painkiller for PMS symptoms. I felt horrible, called in sick to work frequently, and looked awful, wearing anything that would cover the fat. I was moody, irritable, and depressed, which took a toll on my husband and three children.

I started to walk around the mall, and in 5 months, I lost 10 pounds. It was a good start, and I began to feel better. But I hadn't changed my eating habits. Everything I read seemed too hard, too time consuming, or too expensive. I'd tried weight loss plans like Slim-Fast, Elaine Powers, Jenny Craig, Weight Watchers, and numerous fad diets. I never stuck with anything. They just didn't work for me with full-time work and mothering.

When a magazine featuring the South Beach Diet arrived, it literally started a new life for me. After Phase 1, when you "detox" your body, I noticed a huge change in my taste buds. I crave salads now and find them very satisfying. Yogurt tastes extremely sweet and satisfies my sweet tooth. For the first time, I'm really tasting my food and feeling satisfied with a different palate of foods. My cravings for pasta, pastries, and bread have completely disappeared.

So far I'm down to 206 pounds, well on my way to my goal of 135. My clothing has dropped from a size 26 to a size 20. My blood pressure and arthritis meds have been adjusted to almost half of what I was taking. Another positive side effect has been a reduction of the severe PMS symptoms I had been experiencing—surely a combination of the soy I have added to my diet and my new South Beach way of life.

Throughout my weight loss, my family has been so supportive. My 14-year-old is amazed to be able to feel my ribs. My 7-year-old asks, "Can you eat this?" and I respond, "Yes, I could have that, but I'd really rather have this, because it's healthier." She's getting the message early about making better choices. My husband has been wonderful, too, cooking meals when I say I need to go for a walk, which I now do three times a week for 3 to 5 miles.

For the first time, I truly understand the expression "Eat to live, not live to eat." Understanding this is what really changed my mind-set, not to mention my appearance.
—*TERRI L.*

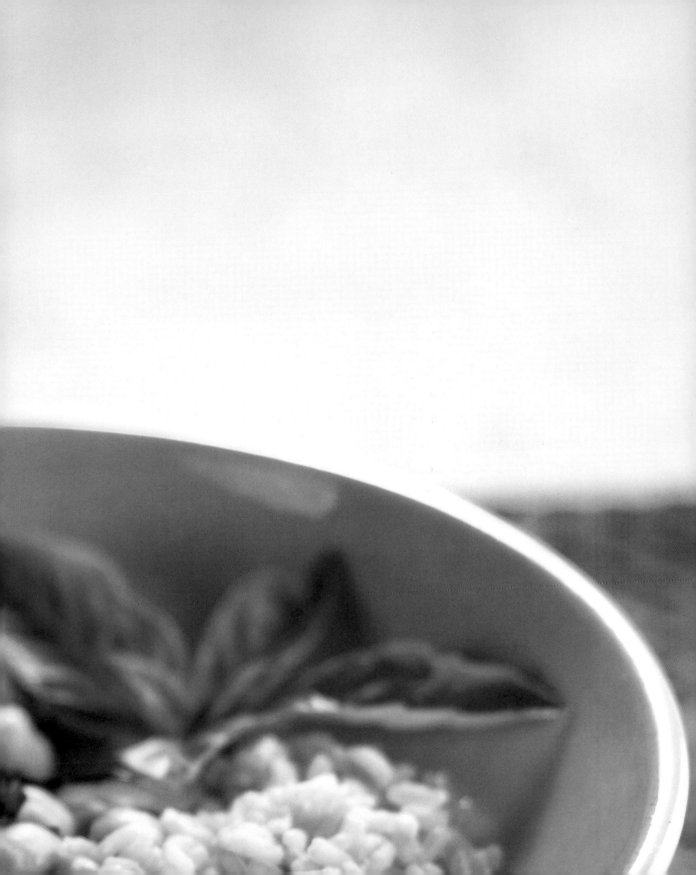

VEGETARIAN ENTRÉES

Even vegetarians sometimes need help with weight control, believe it or not. When you're not getting protein from meat, you tend to rely more heavily on carbs, which can lead to overindulging in some of the wrong kinds. But you can eat well on the South Beach Diet even if you don't include fish or meat in the plan.

Tofu, made from soybeans, is a terrific staple of the vegetarian diet. It's a great source of protein and can be the mainstay of extremely tasty dishes, as this chapter illustrates. The beauty of tofu is how it takes on the flavor of whatever seasonings you use, as in our recipe for Stir-Fry of Broccoli with Tofu and Cherry Tomatoes.

We've also come up with dishes using beans and whole grains, such as barley and brown rice. And there's even a recipe calling for pasta made from spelt, which is an ancient cereal grain that's rich in protein.

Thai Vegetable Stir-Fry

In order to be called Thai, a recipe needs to have all five flavors: Do you taste hot/spicy? Salty? Sweet? Bitter/aromatic? And sour? If so, it's Thai!

- 1 can (14 ounces) light coconut milk (no sugar added)
- 2 cloves garlic, minced
- 1/2 teaspoon grated lemon peel
- 1/2 teaspoon grated lime peel
- 2 cups sliced asparagus tips
- 1 cup halved mushrooms
- 1 small red bell pepper, sliced
- 1 small head bok choy, stems sliced and leaves left whole
- 1/4 cup unsalted peanuts
- 1/2 teaspoon crushed red-pepper flakes
- 1 tablespoon light soy sauce
- 1 tablespoon fresh lime juice
- 1 tablespoon fresh lemon juice
- 1 small bunch fresh basil, slivered

In a food processor, combine the coconut milk, garlic, lemon peel, and lime peel. Pulse to process into a paste. Remove to a large skillet. Place over medium-high heat and cook, stirring, for 1 minute. Add the asparagus, mushrooms, bell pepper, bok choy, peanuts, and red-pepper flakes and simmer for 10 minutes. Stir

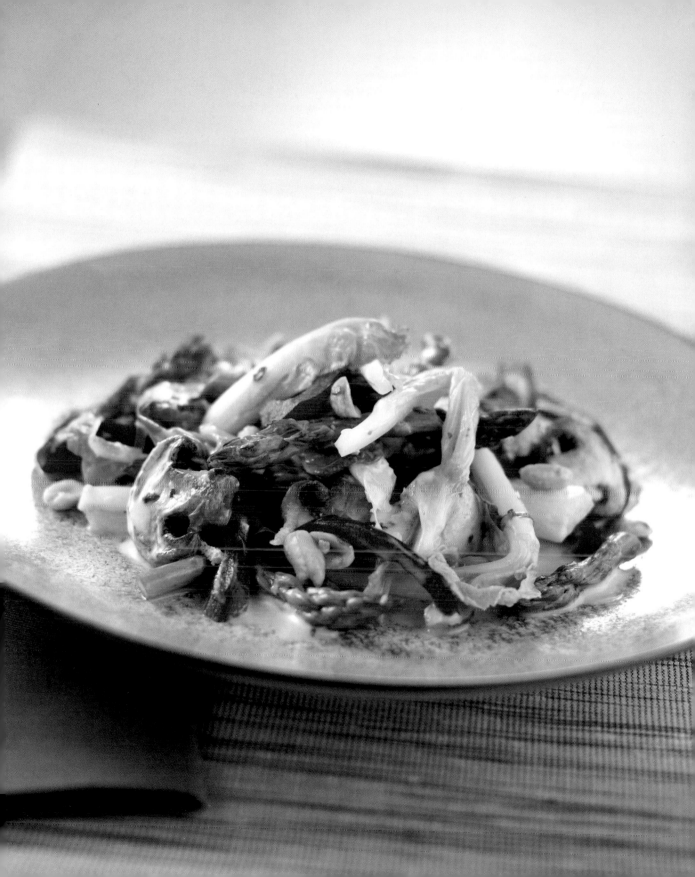

in the soy sauce, lime juice, lemon juice, and basil and simmer, stirring constantly, for 5 minutes.

Makes 4 servings

NUTRITION AT A GLANCE

Per serving: 136 calories, 6 g fat, 1 g saturated fat, 10 g protein, 17 g carbohydrate, 6 g dietary fiber, 0 mg cholesterol, 317 mg sodium

Chickpea Basil Sauté

Chickpeas have been a staple of the Orient and Mediterranean for centuries. They are an excellent source of protein and fiber. This makes a great vegetarian entrée or side with one of the chicken recipes. Without the brown rice, this is a Phase 1 recipe.

1	tablespoon extra virgin olive oil
2	medium onions, sliced
1/2	teaspoon cumin seeds
1	small red bell pepper, cut into strips
1	tablespoon water
3	scallions, chopped
2	cans (14–19 ounces each) chickpeas, rinsed and drained
2	cups chopped fresh basil
2	cups hot cooked brown rice
	Sprig basil, for garnish

Heat the oil in a large nonstick skillet over medium-high heat. Add the onions and cumin seeds and cook, stirring frequently, for 7 minutes. Add the pepper and water. Cover, reduce the heat to low, and cook for 2 minutes. Add the scallions and chickpeas and cook for 2 minutes. Remove from the heat, and add the basil. Serve with the rice. Garnish with the basil.

Makes 4 servings

NUTRITION AT A GLANCE

Per serving: 312 calories, 6 g fat, 1 g saturated fat, 9 g protein, 56 g carbohydrate, 10 g dietary fiber, 0 mg cholesterol, 310 mg sodium

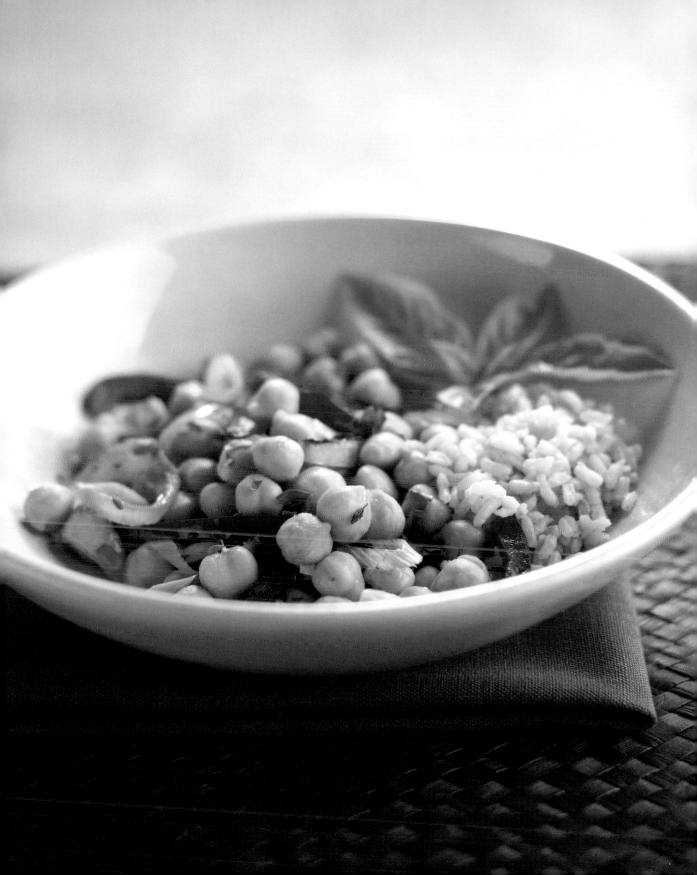

From the Menu of . . .

BLEAU VIEW, FONTAINEBLEAU HILTON RESORT

4441 Collins Avenue, Miami Beach

CHEF BILL ZUPPAS

LOCATED AT ONE OF MIAMI'S BEST-LOVED RESORTS, THE *BLEAU VIEW* COMBINES EUROPEAN AMBIANCE WITH SOUTH BEACH STYLE. THE UPDATED CONTINENTAL FARE, LIKE THIS RISOTTO, RELIES HEAVILY ON MEDITERRANEAN FLAVORS AND SPICES.

Mediterranean Vegetable Risotto with Organic Short-Grain Brown Rice

PHASE 2

2   cups green beans, cut into 1/2 " pieces

2   cups green cabbage, shredded

2   cups organic short-grain brown rice

4   cups water

3   tablespoons extra virgin olive oil

1 onion, finely chopped

1 clove garlic, minced

2 carrots, chopped

2 ribs celery, trimmed and chopped

1 large tomato, seeded and chopped

2 tablespoons chopped parsley

   Sea salt

   Fresh ground black pepper

Bring a saucepan of water to a boil and cook the green beans for 3 to 4 minutes until tender. Add the cabbage and cook for 2 to 3 minutes until tender. Drain the vegetables and set aside.

Put the rice, water, and 1 tablespoon oil in a pot with a tightly fitting lid. Bring to a boil, reduce heat, cover, and simmer for 50 minutes. Remove from the heat and allow to sit, covered, for 10 minutes.

Heat the remaining 2 tablespoons oil in a large skillet. Sauté the onion, garlic, carrots, and celery, until crisp-tender.

Add the tomato, green beans, and cabbage and reheat.

Add the rice and reheat. Remove from the heat and stir in the parsley. Season with salt and pepper to taste.

Makes 8 (side dish) servings

NUTRITION AT A GLANCE

Per serving: 250 calories, 7 g fat, 1 g saturated fat, 5 g protein, 47 g carbohydrate, 5 g dietary fiber, 0 mg cholesterol, 90 mg sodium

Tofu Cacciatore

Cacciatore *means "hunter-style." Because I'm not a hunter, I decided to take solace after a hard day's hunt (work) with tofu instead of pheasant or hare.*

1	pound firm light tofu, cut into 1/2" slices
1/2	medium onion, sliced
1/2	red bell pepper, sliced
1/2	green bell pepper, sliced
2	tablespoons white wine
1	large clove garlic, minced
1	teaspoon dried basil
1	teaspoon dried oregano
	Pinch of allspice
1	can (28 ounces each) stewed tomatoes, drained
2	teaspoons tomato paste
	Sprig rosemary, for garnish

Cover a 17" × 11" baking sheet with paper towels. Place the tofu in a single layer on the towels. Cover the tofu with paper towels and pat down on the tofu until dry. Remove and discard all of the paper towels and place the tofu back on the baking sheet.

Preheat the oven to 350°F.

Heat a large skillet coated with olive oil cooking spray over medium heat. Add the onion and bell peppers and cook, stirring frequently, for 5 minutes. Add the wine, garlic, basil, oregano, and allspice and cook, stirring, for 1 minute. Add the tomatoes and tomato paste. Bring to a boil and allow to simmer for 15 minutes.

Heat another large skillet coated with olive oil cooking spray over medium heat. Add the tofu and sauté for 3 minutes, or until lightly browned on both sides. Place the browned tofu slices in a 13" × 9" baking dish and cover with the tomato sauce.

Bake for 1 hour, or until cooked through. Garnish with the rosemary.

Makes 4 servings

NUTRITION AT A GLANCE
Per serving: 120 calories, 1 g fat, 0 g saturated fat, 10 g protein, 19 g carbohydrate, 3 g dietary fiber, 0 mg cholesterol, 540 mg sodium

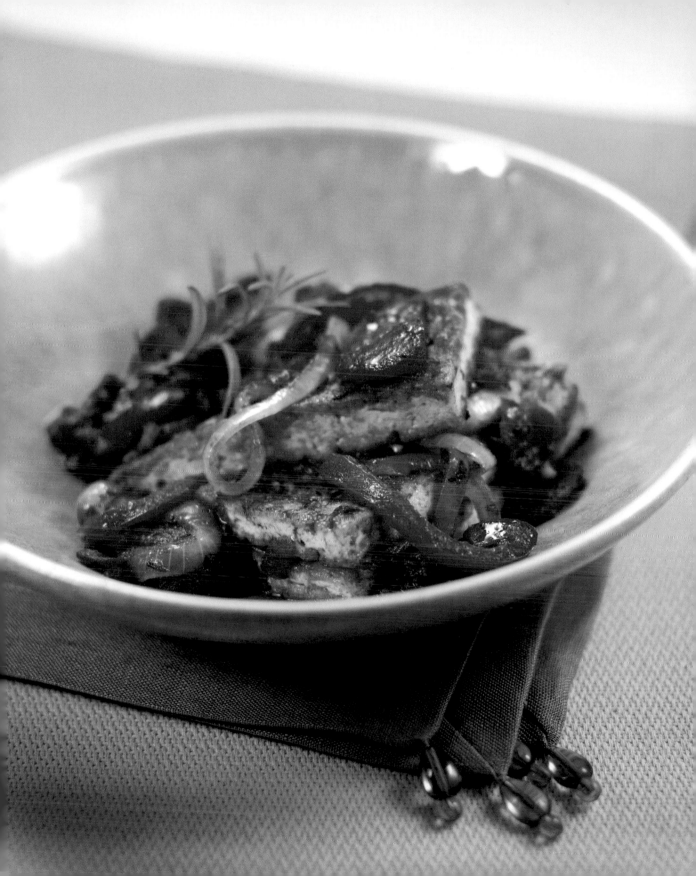

Stir-Fry of Broccoli with Tofu and Cherry Tomatoes

Tofu is a chameleon ingredient that takes on the flavors of the foods that it cooks with. Here, it adopts a sweet-and-sour flavor from garlic, sherry, and soy. Stir-frys cook very quickly, so be sure to have all your ingredients chopped and ready to add to the pan before you begin cooking.

1/3	cup vegetable broth
1	tablespoon light soy sauce
1	tablespoon dry sherry
2	tablespoons cornstarch
1	tablespoon canola oil
1	large bunch broccoli, cut into small florets
4	cloves garlic, minced
1	tablespoon finely chopped fresh ginger
4	ounces mushrooms, sliced
1	cup cherry or yellow pear tomatoes, halved
8	ounces firm tofu, drained and cut into 1/4" cubes

In a cup, whisk together the broth, soy sauce, sherry, and cornstarch. Set aside.

Heat the oil in a large nonstick skillet over medium-high heat. Add the broccoli, garlic, and ginger and cook, stirring constantly, for 1 minute. Add the mushrooms and cook, stirring frequently, for 3 minutes, or until tender and lightly browned.

Add the tomatoes and tofu and cook, stirring frequently, for 2 minutes, or until the tomatoes begin to collapse.

Stir the cornstarch mixture and add to the skillet. Cook, stirring, for 2 minutes, or until the mixture boils and thickens.

Makes 4 servings

NUTRITION AT A GLANCE

Per serving: 151 calories, 8 g fat, 1 g saturated fat, 10 g protein, 13 g carbohydrate, 4 g dietary fiber, 0 mg cholesterol, 195 mg sodium

From the Menu of . . .
CHEF ALLEN'S
19088 NE 29th Avenue, Aventura, Florida

CHEF-PROPRIETOR ALLEN SUSSER

Befitting its sunny South Florida location, *Chef Allen's* serves what Chef-Proprietor Allen Susser calls "Palm Tree Cuisine." It's a kind of global thinking about food and recipes that, as he puts it, "encourages the fusing of ingredients of many cuisines and cultures."

Caribbean Ratatouille
PHASE 3

2 tablespoons extra virgin olive oil

1 large onion, chopped

1 small green plantain, chopped

1 cup chopped calabaza

2 medium chayote, chopped

2 medium Anaheim chiles, seeded and chopped

1 medium red bell pepper, seeded and chopped

1/2 tablespoon chopped garlic

1 teaspoon oregano

1   teaspoon cumin

1   teaspoon ground black peppercorns

1   tablespoon kosher salt

1   cup freshly squeezed orange juice

In a large Dutch oven, warm the olive oil. Add the onion and cook until translucent. Then add each of the vegetables at 2-minute intervals, starting with the plantain, calabaza, chayote, Anaheim chile, and red pepper. Stir well but try not to crush any of the vegetables.

Season with the garlic, oregano, cumin, peppercorns, and salt. Moisten the mixture with orange juice. Simmer for 5 minutes, or until tender, allowing all the flavors to incorporate yet not lose the integrity of each vegetable.

Makes 4 servings

NUTRITION AT A GLANCE

Per serving: 203 calories, 7 g fat, 1 g saturated fat, 3 g protein, 35 g carbohydrate, 6 g dietary fiber, 0 mg cholesterol, 1,172 mg sodium

Tofu with Salsa

The habañero chile pepper gives you lots of flavor—and quite a bit of heat. If you want to fire things up even more, replace it with a couple of tepín chile peppers. Smoked tofu is one of the tastiest of tofu products, but each brand tastes different, so you will have to experiment to see which one you like the best.

1/2	pound smoked tofu, cut into 8 thin slices
1	large beefsteak tomato, skinned, seeded, and finely chopped
1/4	cup extra virgin olive oil
1	clove garlic, minced
2	tablespoons chopped parsley
1	small habañero chile pepper, seeded and finely chopped (wear plastic gloves when handling)
1	teaspoon red wine vinegar
1/4	teaspoon sugar substitute

Place the tofu in a single layer in a shallow dish.

In a small bowl combine the tomato, oil, garlic, parsley, chile pepper, vinegar, and sugar substitute and whisk to blend well.

Spoon the salsa mixture over the tofu and allow to marinate for 30 minutes.

Serve 2 slices of tofu per plate topped with the salsa.

Makes 4 servings

NUTRITION AT A GLANCE

Per serving: 258 calories, 20 g fat, 3 g saturated fat, 13 g protein, 6 g carbohydrate, 1 g dietary fiber, 0 mg cholesterol, 245 mg sodium

Spinach Dumplings

These cheesy dumplings are topped off with a little nutmeg.

> 2 packages (8 ounces each) frozen chopped spinach
>
> 2 teaspoons salt
>
> 2 eggs
>
> 1 2/3 cups whole wheat bread crumbs
>
> 1 teaspoon Italian seasoning
>
> 2/3 pound reduced-fat ricotta cheese
>
> 1/4 cup (1 ounce) grated Parmesan cheese
>
> 3 scallions, minced
>
> 1/3 cup chopped parsley
>
> 2 teaspoons finely chopped fresh basil
>
> 1 clove garlic, minced
>
> Pinch of ground nutmeg
>
> Pinch of ground black pepper
>
> Whole wheat flour
>
> 4–6 quarts water
>
> South Beach Tomato Sauce (see page 234)

In a medium saucepan over low heat, combine the spinach and 1 1/2 teaspoons of the salt. Cover and cook the spinach for 15 minutes, or until completely thawed. Drain. Use your hands to squeeze out as much water as possible.

Beat the eggs in a large bowl. Add the spinach, bread crumbs, Italian seasoning, ricotta cheese, Parmesan cheese, scallions, parsley, basil, garlic, nutmeg, and pepper. Mix well, then cover and refrigerate for 24 hours.

Preheat the oven to 250°F.

Form the mixture, 1/3 cup at a time, into oval dumplings, about 3" long and 1 1/2 " wide. Roll each dumpling in flour. Do not allow the dumplings to touch each other as you finish them.

Bring the water and the remaining 1/2 teaspoon salt to a boil in a large pot over medium-high heat. Drop enough dumplings into the water to make one layer. When the dumplings float to the surface, cook for an additional 4 minutes. Remove the dumplings with a slotted spoon, draining well.

Coat an ovenproof dish with olive oil cooking spray. Place the dumplings in the dish and place in the oven. Cook the remaining dumplings in the same manner. When all the dumplings are in the oven, warm the tomato sauce in a medium saucepan over medium-low heat.

Evenly divide the dumplings among 4 serving dishes and top with the tomato sauce. Serve additional sauce on the side.

Makes 4 servings

NUTRITION AT A GLANCE

Per serving: 290 calories, 15 g fat, 9 g saturated fat, 20 g protein, 19 g carbohydrate, 5 g dietary fiber, 150 mg cholesterol, 1,000 mg sodium

Arugula and Basil Pesto Linguine

Spelt is a high-protein ancient grain that's enjoying a resurgence. This flavorful pasta is perfect for a cold night's supper.

12	ounces spelt linguine
4	cups arugula leaves
1	cup tightly packed basil leaves
3–4	cloves garlic, minced
2	tablespoons pine nuts
	Salt
	Ground black pepper
1/3	cup extra virgin olive oil
1/4	cup grated Parmesan cheese

Prepare the pasta according to package directions. Drain and place in a large serving bowl.

Meanwhile, in a food processor, combine the arugula, basil, garlic, pine nuts, and salt and pepper to taste. Process to coarsely chop.

With the food processor running, slowly add the oil in a steady stream until the mixture is smooth.

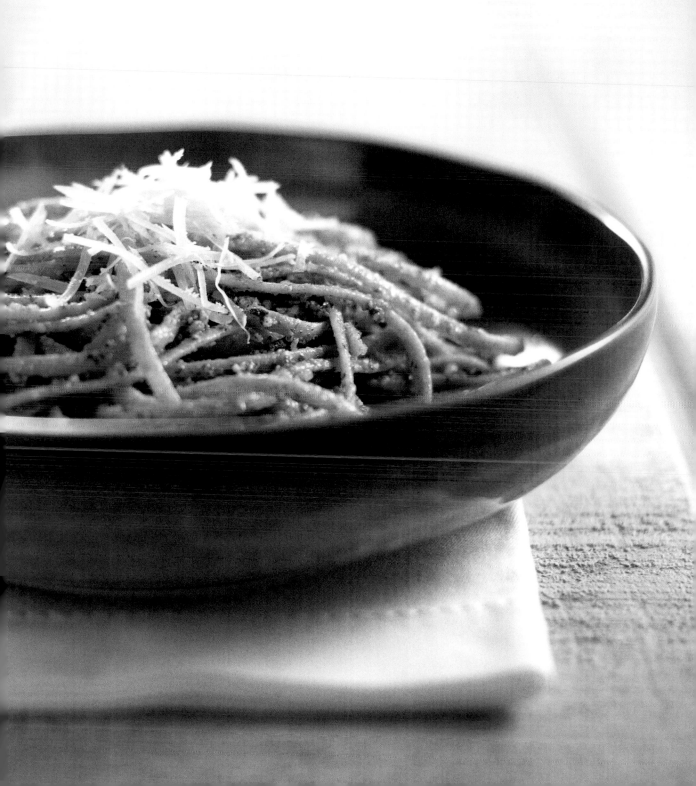

Toss the pasta with the pesto. Sprinkle with the cheese.

Makes 4 servings

NUTRITION AT A GLANCE

Per serving: 520 calories, 21 g fat, 3 1/2 g saturated fat, 17 g protein, 65 g carbohydrate, 4 g dietary fiber, 5 mg cholesterol, 100 mg sodium

I'M FOCUSING ON MAKING MEALS THAT ARE AESTHETICALLY PLEASING AND BEAUTIFUL TO LOOK AT.

I'm 47 years old and single. I'd always enjoyed a healthy, active lifestyle and felt great until last year, when an unexpected hysterectomy got me off track emotionally and physically. I stopped exercising, ate the wrong things, and gained about 50 pounds while recovering from surgery. My doctor made it clear that if I didn't start making changes, I was headed toward diabetes.

I started with Weight Watchers. It was convenient because we had weekly meetings at work. Then I heard about South Beach, and now I am doing a kind of hybrid approach: eating the South Beach way, and receiving emotional support through my WW group.

With this combination, I've lost 60 pounds so far, but have not yet reached my goal of wearing clothes smaller than a size 12. For me, slow and steady has been key. I like the structure of the SB plan. Deprivation equals bingeing, in my experience, and this diet allows you the things you want. Before South Beach, I was the kind of person who could eat a whole loaf of French bread. Now I can have a piece of French bread if I want to, but my meals are more balanced.

Another thing that has helped is focusing on making meals that are aesthetically pleasing and beautiful to look at. I've become very fond of vegetables—their colors and textures are amazing! I'm more visually aware of food. When I've created something beautiful to look at, I savor it—no more cramming!

Eating out is often a challenge, but I have found that telling people I have dietary restrictions garners more respect than saying I am on a diet. I am not shy about asking for substitutions, and I ask that they bring a takeout container to the table when they bring the meal, so that I can immediately save half for later.

For me, weight control has shifted from wanting to be model-thin or attract a certain type of man, to wanting to maintain a healthy BMI (body mass index), to avoid obesity-related conditions such as diabetes, and to live a long life. Life is a gift, and keeping myself in shape is the best gift that I can give to myself. —*SUSAN W.*

Whole Wheat Vegetable Lasagna

This dish can be enjoyed right away, but like many casseroles, it tastes even better the next day.

- 1 teaspoon extra virgin olive oil
- 1 zucchini, sliced
- 2 cups (16 ounces) reduced-fat ricotta cheese
- 1 egg
- 1 tablespoon dried basil
- 1/4 teaspoon salt
- 1/8 teaspoon ground black pepper
- 2 cups South Beach Tomato Sauce (see page 234) or low-sugar spaghetti sauce
- 9 whole wheat lasagna noodles, cooked
- 1 package (10 ounces) frozen chopped spinach, thawed and squeezed dry
- 1/4 cup (1 ounce) grated Parmesan cheese
- 1/4 cup (1 ounce) shredded reduced-fat mozzarella cheese

Preheat the oven to 350°F. Coat a 13" × 9" baking dish with cooking spray.

Heat the oil in a medium skillet over medium heat. Add the zucchini and cook for 5 minutes, or until crisp-tender. Remove from the heat and set aside.

In a medium bowl, combine the ricotta, egg, basil, salt, and pepper. Set aside 1/2 cup of the spaghetti sauce.

Place 3 lasagna noodles in the prepared baking dish. Evenly spoon half of the spaghetti sauce over the noodles. Top with half of the ricotta mixture, half of the spinach, half of the zucchini, and half of the Parmesan. Repeat layering with 3 more noodles and the remaining ingredients. End with the remaining 3 noodles. Spoon the remaining sauce over top and sprinkle with the mozzarella.

Cover with foil and bake for 25 minutes. Uncover and bake for 20 minutes longer, or until hot and bubbly. Let stand for 10 minutes before serving.

Makes 12 servings

NUTRITION AT A GLANCE

Per serving: 217 calories, 7 g fat, 4 g saturated fat, 12 g protein, 29 g carbohydrate, 4 g dietary fiber, 44 mg cholesterol, 36 mg sodium

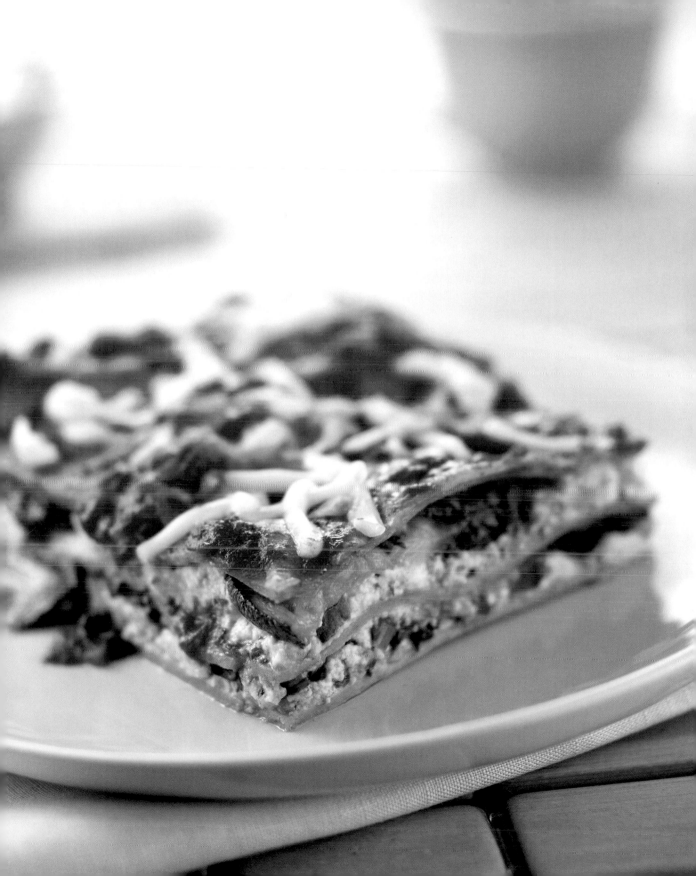

From the Menu of . . .
MACALUSO'S
1747 Alton Road, Miami Beach

CHEF MICHAEL D'ANDREA

Escarole and beans is a classic Italian dish that's right at home at this friendly *trattoria*, a favorite of Miami Beach locals.

Macaluso's Escarole and Beans
PHASE 1

1/4	cup extra virgin olive oil
5	cloves garlic, minced
1/2	teaspoon salt
1/2	teaspoon pepper
	Pinch of crushed red-pepper flakes
3	heads escarole, cut into 2–3" pieces
1/2	can Progresso white cannellini beans, undrained
2	tablespoons Percorino Romano cheese (optional)

In a large pot, heat the oil, garlic, salt, pepper, and red-pepper flakes over medium heat. Do not let the garlic brown. Add the escarole and stir until halfway cooked. Add the beans with juice. Raise the heat to medium-high, just long enough to heat the beans, about 1 to 2 minutes.

Remove the pot from the heat. Add the cheese, if using.

Makes 4 servings

NUTRITION AT A GLANCE

Per serving: 210 calories, 11 g fat, 1 1/2 g saturated fat, 8 g protein, 23 g carbohydrate, 11 g dietary fiber, 0 mg cholesterol, 350 mg sodium

Vegetarian Chili with Avocado Salsa

This flavor-packed chili will leave you wondering where you could put any meat, even if you wanted it.

Avocado Salsa

- 1 medium California avocado, peeled, pitted, and finely chopped
- 1 small tomato, finely chopped
- 1/4 red onion, finely chopped
- 1 clove garlic, minced
- 1 tablespoon chopped fresh cilantro
- Juice of 1 large lime
- 1/4 teaspoon ground cumin
- 1/4 teaspoon ground black pepper

Vegetarian Chili

- 2 teaspoons extra virgin olive oil
- 1 onion, chopped
- 1 red bell pepper, chopped
- 3/4 can (14–19 ounces) black beans, rinsed and drained
- 3/4 can (14 1/2 ounces) diced tomatoes
- 3/4 can (14 ounces) vegetable broth
- 1 can (4 ounces) green chile peppers, chopped
- 2 teaspoons chili powder
- 2 cloves garlic, minced
- 1 teaspoon ground cumin

             1 teaspoon dried oregano

         1/4   cup fat-free sour cream

             1 lime, quartered

             2 tablespoons chopped fresh cilantro

           12   whole wheat pita crisps (Phase 2 or 3)

To make the avocado salsa: In a large bowl, combine the avocado, tomato, onion, garlic, cilantro, lime juice, cumin, and pepper. Lightly toss. Let stand for 30 minutes.

To make the vegetarian chili: Meanwhile, heat the oil in a 6-quart Dutch oven over medium-high heat. Add the onion and bell pepper and cook, stirring frequently, for 3 minutes. Add the beans, tomatoes (with juice), broth, chile peppers, chili powder, garlic, cumin, and oregano and simmer for 20 minutes. Serve with the avocado salsa, sour cream, and lime wedges. Sprinkle with the cilantro. Serve the pita crisps on the side, if using.

Makes 6 servings

NUTRITION AT A GLANCE

Per serving: 181 calories, 17 g fat, 1 g saturated fat, 7 g protein, 25 g carbohydrate, 15 g dietary fiber, 0 mg cholesterol, 665 mg sodium

Barley with Mushrooms

The meaty and full-flavored mushrooms combine with the nuttiness from the barley and cheese to make this a true winner.

1/2	ounce dried porcini mushrooms
1	cup hot water
3	tablespoons extra virgin olive oil
4	cloves garlic, minced
6	ounces portobello mushroom caps, chopped
1	bunch scallions, finely chopped
2	cans vegetable broth
1	cup medium pearl barley
	Salt
	Ground black pepper
1/2	cup (2 ounces) grated Romano cheese
1/4	cup (1 ounce) grated Parmesan cheese

In a large bowl, combine the porcini mushrooms with the hot water. Set aside.

Heat the oil in a large skillet over medium-high heat. Add the garlic and portobello mushrooms and cook, stirring occasionally, for 10 minutes, or until they begin to brown. Drain the porcini mushrooms, then cut into small pieces and add to the skillet. Cook for 1 minute. Add 2 tablespoons of the scallions, the broth, barley, and salt and pepper to taste. Bring to almost a boil. Reduce the heat to low, cover, and simmer for 12 minutes, or until almost all of the liquid is absorbed. Remove from the heat and add the Romano. Just before serving, add the remaining scallions and sprinkle with the Parmesan.

Makes 4 servings

NUTRITION AT A GLANCE

Per serving: 389 calories, 16 g fat, 4 1/2 g saturated fat, 13 g protein, 45 g carbohydrate, 9 g dietary fiber, 15 mg cholesterol, 610 mg sodium

Garlic and Lemon Grilled Vegetables

Grilled vegetables are always a special treat. Give the veggies a little time to marinate to soak up lots of extra flavor. If you like, you can even prepare them a day or two beforehand, then cook them up quickly when you're ready.

1/4	cup chopped flat-leaf parsley
3	tablespoons lemon juice
2	tablespoons extra virgin olive oil
3	cloves garlic, minced
1	teaspoon dried Italian seasoning
1/2	teaspoon ground black pepper
1/4	teaspoon salt
2	large roasted red peppers, cut into strips
6	ounces portobello mushrooms, sliced
1	large purple onion, halved and cut into 1"-thick slices

Coat a grill rack with cooking spray. Preheat the grill to medium-hot.

In a large bowl, combine the parsley, lemon juice, oil, garlic, Italian seasoning, black pepper, and salt. Add the roasted peppers, mushrooms, and onion and toss to coat well. (The mixture can be prepared ahead to this point and refrigerated for up to 2 days.)

Place a vegetable basket or grill screen on the grill rack and place the vegetables on the basket or screen.

Grill, turning often, for 15 minutes, or until very tender and lightly charred.

Makes 4 servings

Baked Portobello Caps with Melted Goat Cheese

For a super lunch or supper, serve these delicious caps with a fresh green salad.

> 1 cup South Beach Tomato Sauce (see page 234) or low-sugar spaghetti sauce
>
> 4 large portobello mushroom caps
>
> 1 package (4 ounces) reduced-fat goat cheese, cut into 4 pieces
>
> 2 tablespoons pine nuts, finely chopped
>
> 1 tablespoon chopped fresh basil
>
> Sprig basil, for garnish

Preheat the oven to 375°F.

Spread the sauce in the bottom of a 9" × 9" baking dish. Arrange the mushroom caps, gill side up, on top. Place a piece of goat cheese on each mushroom. Sprinkle evenly with the pine nuts.

Bake for 30 minutes, or until hot and bubbly. Top with the chopped basil. Garnish with the basil sprig.

Makes 4 servings

NUTRITION AT A GLANCE

Per serving: 190 calories, 13 g fat, 3 1/2 g saturated fat, 9 g protein, 9 g carbohydrate, 3 g dietary fiber, 10 mg cholesterol, 590 mg sodium

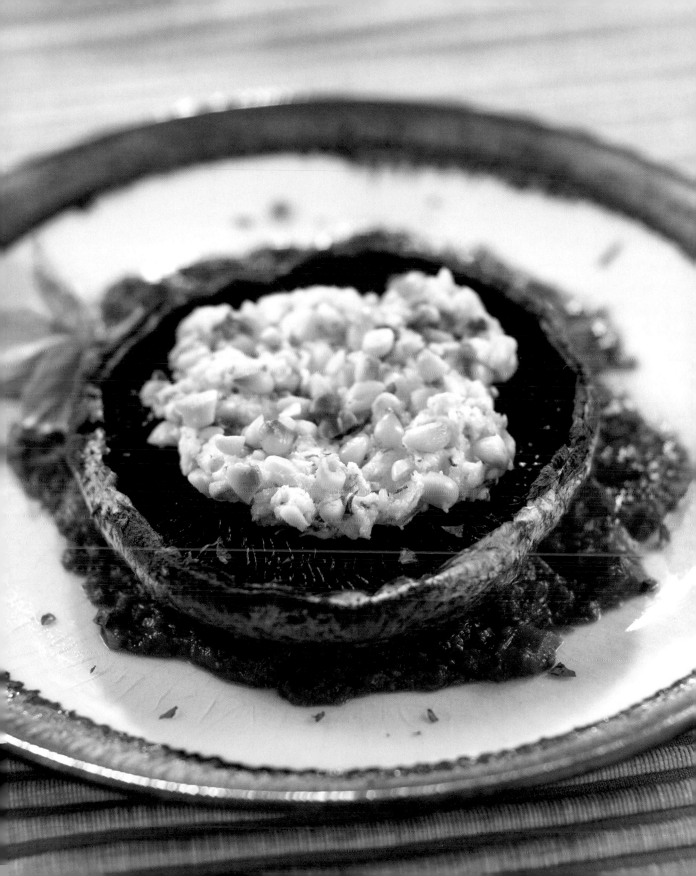

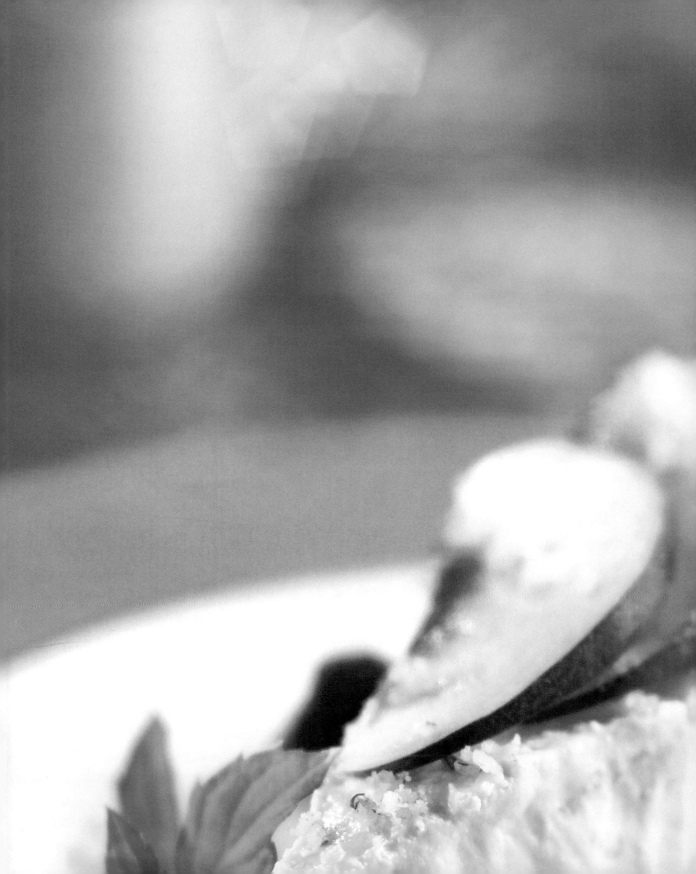

DESSERTS

As I pointed out earlier in this book, I am a chocoholic. That may have something to do with the fact that the South Beach Diet allows you to eat dessert. Our reasoning is simple: A good diet should strive to allow you to eat normally, and for most people, that means having something sweet to top off a good meal. We've tried hard to devise some great desserts that keep to the diet so that you don't have to cheat in order to satisfy your sweet tooth. The truth is, if you use a sugar substitute instead of the real thing, you'll be doing yourself a great favor without sacrificing anything on taste. Stick with goodies like dark chocolate, fruit, and cheese, and steer clear of desserts made from white flour or other processed carbs, and you can indulge on a daily basis and still lose weight.

Chilled Espresso Custard

Complement your meal with coffee at its best—a simply lovely baked custard of rich-tasting espresso.

1 1/2 cups 1% milk

2 eggs, beaten

3 tablespoons sugar substitute

2 teaspoons espresso powder or instant decaffeinated coffee

1 teaspoon vanilla extract

Ground cinnamon, for garnish

Lemon twists, for garnish

In a medium bowl, whisk together the milk, eggs, sugar substitute, espresso powder or coffee, and vanilla extract until well-blended. Pour into four 6-ounce custard cups or ramekins and place in a 10" skillet.

Fill the skillet with water to 1/2" from the tops of the custard cups. Bring the water to a boil over high heat. Reduce the heat to low, cover, and simmer for 10 minutes. Remove the cups from the skillet, cover with plastic wrap touching the surface of the pudding, and refrigerate for 3 hours, or until chilled. Garnish with the cinnamon and lemon twists.

Makes 4 servings

NUTRITION AT A GLANCE

Per serving: 110 calories, 3 1/2 g fat, 1 1/2 g saturated fat, 6 g protein, 13 g carbohydrate, 0 g dietary fiber, 110 mg cholesterol, 80 mg sodium

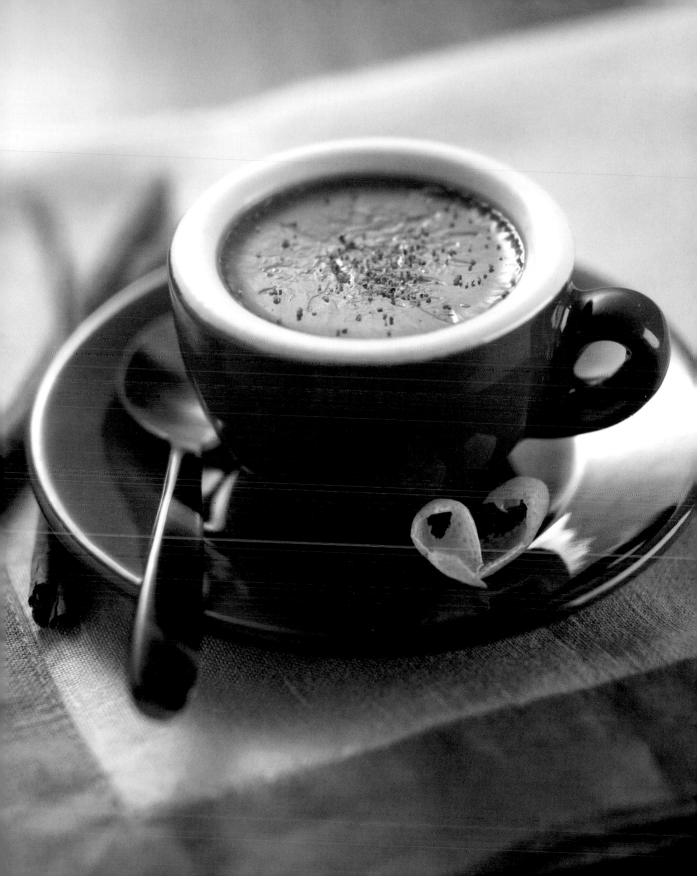

Ricotta Romanoff Sundae

Whether this dessert was first served to the Russian Czar Nicholas I by Marie Careme can be debated, but there is little doubt that you will be glad we came up with this version.

- 2 cups quartered strawberries
- 1 tablespoon grated orange peel
- 3 tablespoons sugar substitute
- 1 1/4 cups sliced strawberries
- 4 cups reduced-fat ricotta cheese
- 2 tablespoons pistachios
- Mint leaves, for garnish

In a blender or food processor, combine the quartered strawberries, orange peel, and sugar substitute and blend until smooth. Pour into a large bowl. Gently stir in the sliced strawberries. Cover and chill.

When ready to serve, evenly divide the ricotta among 4 serving bowls. Pour equal amounts of the strawberry mixture over the ricotta, then sprinkle with the pistachios. Garnish with the mint leaves.

Makes 8 servings

NUTRITION AT A GLANCE

Per serving: 220 calories, 11 g fat, 6 g saturated fat, 15 g protein, 15 g carbohydrate, 2 g dietary fiber, 40 mg cholesterol, 160 mg sodium

Strawberries with Velvety Chocolate Dip

Strawberries with chocolate dip are so easy to prepare, yet they have a wonderfully fancy feel. For a special presentation, serve the dip in a clear crystal bowl on a platter circled with the strawberries.

6 tablespoons fat-free plain yogurt

6 tablespoons sugar-free chocolate syrup

1 teaspoon thawed frozen orange juice concentrate

2 pints medium strawberries, hulled

In a small bowl with an electric mixer on medium speed, whip the yogurt, chocolate syrup, and orange juice concentrate. Cover and chill until ready to serve. Serve with the strawberries for dipping.

Makes 6 servings

NUTRITION AT A GLANCE

Per serving: 130 calories, 1/2 g fat, 0 g saturated fat, 3 g protein, 31 g carbohydrate, 4 g dietary fiber, 0 mg cholesterol, 45 mg sodium

Wonton Cups with Fresh Berries

Wonton wrappers are available in the refrigerated produce section of most supermarkets. If you're in a hurry, you can replace the wonton wrappers with prepared phyllo shells from the freezer case of your supermarket.

- 24 wonton wrappers
- 2 tablespoons trans-free margarine, melted
- 1/3 cup sugar-free strawberry preserves
- 1 cup artificially sweetened nonfat lemon yogurt
- 1 1/4 cups fresh blackberries, blueberries, or raspberries

Preheat the oven to 350°F.

Using a 12-cup nonstick muffin pan, line each cup with a wonton wrapper. Brush the wonton wrappers with a little of the margarine. Place second wrappers diagonally on top of each of the first ones, making sure that the points of the wrappers make sides to the cup. Brush the second layer of wrappers with a little margarine.

Bake for 8 minutes, or until golden brown. Cool. Remove from the pan.

Evenly divide the all-fruit spread among the wonton cups.

Place the yogurt in a medium bowl and fold in 1 cup of the berries. Evenly divide the yogurt mixture among the wonton cups. Top with the remaining 1/4 cup berries.

Makes 12 servings

NUTRITION AT A GLANCE

Per serving: 80 calories, 2 g fat, 0 g saturated fat, 3 g protein, 14 g carbohydrate, 1 g dietary fiber, 0 mg cholesterol, 120 mg sodium

Black Cherry Baked Apples

This treat is as simple as it is unusual and delicious.

> 4 baking apples
> 1/2 teaspoon cinnamon
> 1/4 cup dried cherries or raisins
> 1/4 cup walnuts, chopped
> 1 cup diet black cherry soda

Preheat the oven to 375°F.

Using an apple corer or sharp knife, remove the apple cores from the stem ends without cutting the apples all the way through the outer end. Place the apples cored side up in a 9" × 9" baking dish.

Sprinkle the apples inside and outside with the cinnamon. Spoon the cherries or raisins and the walnuts into the apples. Drizzle a little soda into each apple. Pour the remaining soda into the baking dish.

Bake for 20 minutes, or until the apples are tender.

Makes 4 servings

NUTRITION AT A GLANCE

Per serving: 131 calories, 5 g fat, 0 g saturated fat, 1 g protein, 23 g carbohydrate, 4 g dietary fiber, 0 mg cholesterol, 10 mg sodium

Berry Granita

Deliciously refreshing, this is the perfect dessert to serve after a summer meal.

> 1/2 cup water
>
> 1/4 cup sugar substitute
>
> 1 bag (10 ounces) frozen blueberries
>
> 1 lemon, peeled and juiced
>
> Lemon twist, for garnish
>
> 1/2 cup low-fat frozen whipped topping, thawed (optional)

In a small pot over medium heat, combine the water and sugar substitute. Bring to a boil. Boil for 2 minutes, then set aside to cool to room temperature.

In a food processor fitted with a metal blade, combine the blueberries, lemon peel, lemon juice, and cooled syrup. Pulse for 2 minutes, or until the blueberries are coarsely ground. Pour into a small metal bowl and stir a few times with a fork to break up any large pieces. Cover the bowl with foil and place in the freezer overnight.

Spoon into 6 serving glasses, garnish with a lemon twist, and top with the whipped topping, if using.

Makes 6 servings

NUTRITION AT A GLANCE

Per serving: 60 calories, 1/2 g fat, 1/2 g saturated fat, 0 g protein, 14 g carbohydrate, 1 g dietary fiber, 0 mg cholesterol, 0 mg sodium

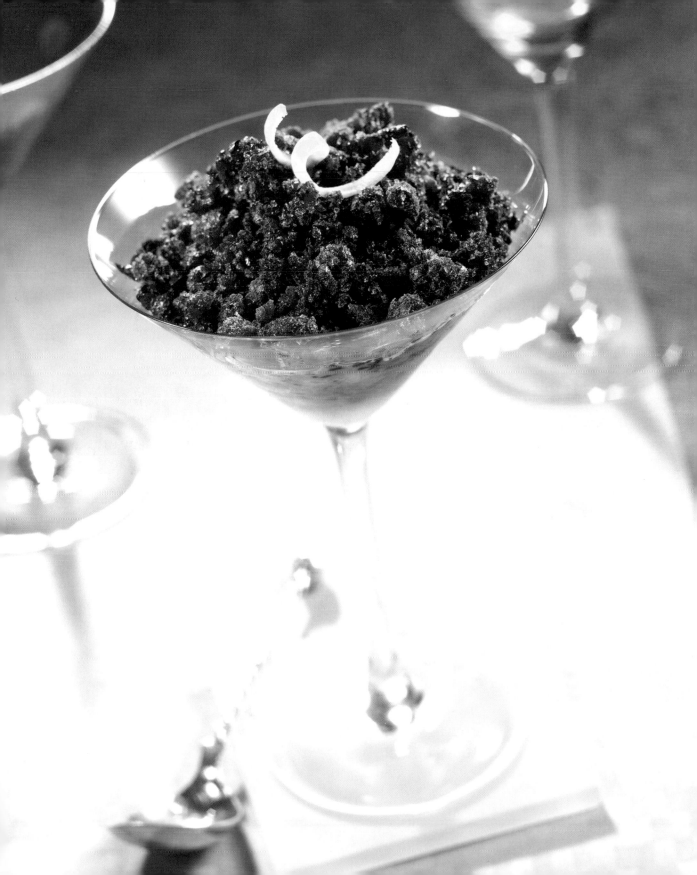

Frozen Strawberry Dessert

Use the berry of your choice, but whatever you do, don't leave this dessert out of your regular rotation.

> 2 tablespoons mayonnaise
>
> 8 ounces reduced-fat cream cheese, softened
>
> 1 tablespoon lemon juice
>
> 1 package (10 ounces) frozen unsweetened strawberries, partially thawed
>
> 1 cup low-fat frozen whipped topping, thawed

In a medium bowl, gradually blend the mayonnaise and the cream cheese and mix well. Add the lemon juice and strawberries, 1/4 cup at a time. Fold in the whipped topping. Evenly divide the mixture into 6 fluted molds and freeze for 2 hours, or until firm. Serve as a sweet dessert salad.

Makes 6 servings

NUTRITION AT A GLANCE

Per serving: 160 calories, 12 g fat, 6 g saturated fat, 4 g protein, 10 g carbohydrate, 1 g dietary fiber, 25 mg cholesterol, 140 mg sodium

Strawberry Buttermilk Ice

Is there anyone who doesn't like something smooth and cold on a warm evening?

> 1 cup sugar substitute
>
> 1 cup water
>
> 2 1/2 cups quartered strawberries
> (about 3 cups whole berries)
>
> 1 cup buttermilk

In a large bowl, combine the sugar substitute and water. In a blender or food processor, blend the strawberries until smooth. Add the strawberries and buttermilk to the sugar substitute mixture and stir until well-combined. Pour into a freezer-safe container. Freeze overnight. Remove from the freezer 30 minutes before serving.

Makes 4 servings

NUTRITION AT A GLANCE

Per serving: 120 calories, 1/2 g fat, 0 g saturated fat, 2 g protein, 27 g carbohydrate, 1 g dietary fiber, 5 mg cholesterol, 45 mg sodium

Strawberry Shimmer

*After succeeding with the South Beach Diet, this will be the
only thing you see shaking when you walk to the table.*

> 1 package (3 ounces) sugar-free strawberry-flavored
> gelatin
>
> 1 cup boiling water
>
> 1 package (10 ounces) frozen unsweetened
> strawberries
>
> 8 ounces artificially sweetened nonfat strawberry
> yogurt

Coat a 4-cup mold with cooking spray.

In a small bowl, dissolve the gelatin in the boiling
water. Add the strawberries and stir until the
strawberries thaw. Chill for 30 minutes, or until
thickened. Beat with an electric mixer on medium
speed until frothy. Fold in the yogurt. Pour the mixture
into the prepared mold and chill for 1 1/2 hours, or
until firm.

Makes 4 servings

NUTRITION AT A GLANCE

Per serving: 70 calories, 0 g fat, 0 g saturated fat, 3 g protein,
14 g carbohydrate, 1 g dietary fiber, 0 mg cholesterol, 40 mg sodium

MY SOUTH BEACH DIET

JUST CALL ME "THE INCREDIBLE SHRINKING GRANNY."

Two months ago, I weighed in at my doctor's office at 342 pounds—the heaviest I have ever been. That night I got an e-mail about the South Beach Diet, and I almost deleted it. Luckily, I visited the Prevention.com Web site, and the rest is history.

By the end of Phase 1, I had lost 19 pounds. In Phase 2, I have been losing about 1/2 pound a day. I haven't cheated yet, and I don't think I will. I am currently down 35 1/2 pounds in only 61 days! I don't exercise yet, but I plan to start once I drop below 300 pounds.

What's great is that almost anything is allowed after the first 2 weeks. Even in Phase 1, the meals and snacks are plentiful. I was never hungry. I have always cooked lunch and dinner, so it wasn't that hard for me to switch from my regular cooking to South Beach cooking.

Recently, at a birthday party for my 6-year-old custodial granddaughter, I had 3 bites of a piece of cake. Afterward, I had a horrible time with cravings for about 24 hours. I wanted chips and cake and cookies and on and on. Luckily, I was able to fill myself up with legal foods, and once I got through that day, I was back on track. That's one way to learn the difference between giving your body the wrong or right fuels.

In the past, I've struggled with chronic health problems like rheumatoid arthritis, chronic fatigue, and fibromyalgia. Since starting the South Beach Diet, I have twice as much energy, and my cholesterol has dropped from 274 to 187. I am able to do so much more with less joint pain. I spend less time resting and more time volunteering at my granddaughter's school. She is so proud that I can be there—a real side benefit I wasn't expecting!

At my recent yearly physical, my doctor said she was impressed enough to go and buy the book and read it for her other patients. She checked my records twice to be sure that the weight recorded 2 months ago was correct. This is really a way of life, not a quick fix. With my online SB support group, I call myself "the Incredible Shrinking Granny." When I'm down to 170 pounds, I'm going to be proud to share who I really am with my granddaughter. I need all the energy and health I can get to keep up with her! —*APRIL G.*

Apple and Almond Soufflé

This is another very light and fluffy treat for dessert lovers out there. You'll notice that almonds have been included for some heart-healthy fat.

3	medium baking apples, peeled, cored, and cut into bite-size pieces
1/4	cup water
3	tablespoons sugar substitute
1/2	teaspoon almond extract
5	egg whites
1/4	cup sliced almonds, toasted (optional)

In a 2-quart saucepan, combine the apples and water. Bring to a boil over high heat. Reduce the heat to low, cover, and simmer, stirring occasionally, for 10 minutes, or until the apples are tender. Stir in the sugar substitute and almond extract. Remove from the heat and place in the refrigerator for 10 minutes. (Place a hot pad underneath the pot in the refrigerator.)

Preheat the oven to 425°F.

In a large bowl, with an electric mixer on high speed, beat the egg whites until stiff peaks form. With a rubber spatula, gently fold into the cooled apple mixture. Spoon the mixture into a 1 1/2-quart soufflé dish.

Bake for 15 minutes, or until the soufflé is puffed and browned. Sprinkle with the almonds before serving, if using. Serve warm.

Makes 4 servings

NUTRITION AT A GLANCE

Per serving: 150 calories, 3 1/2 g fat, 0 g saturated fat, 6 g protein, 25 g carbohydrate, 2 g dietary fiber, 0 mg cholesterol, 70 mg sodium

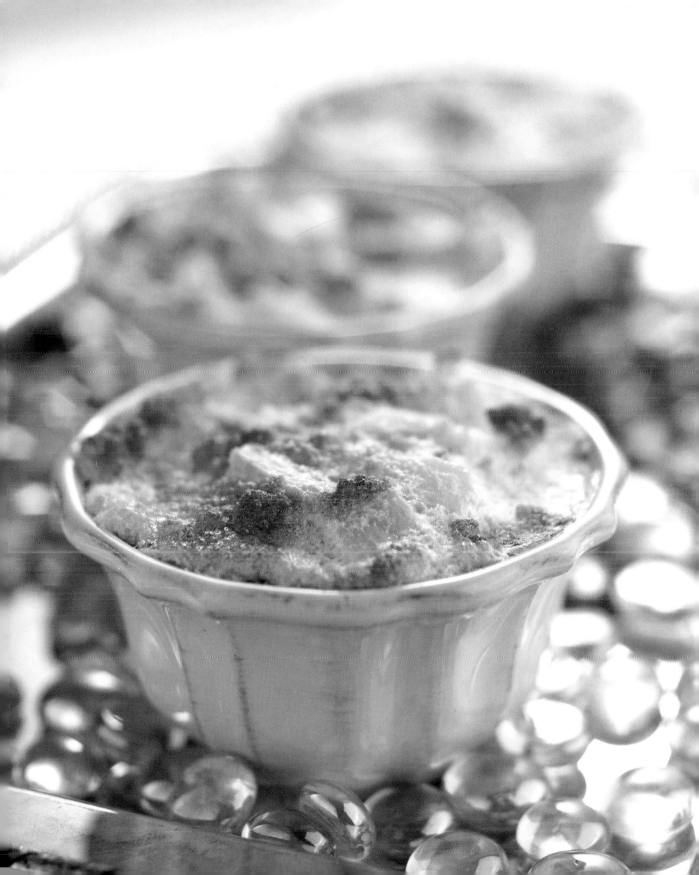

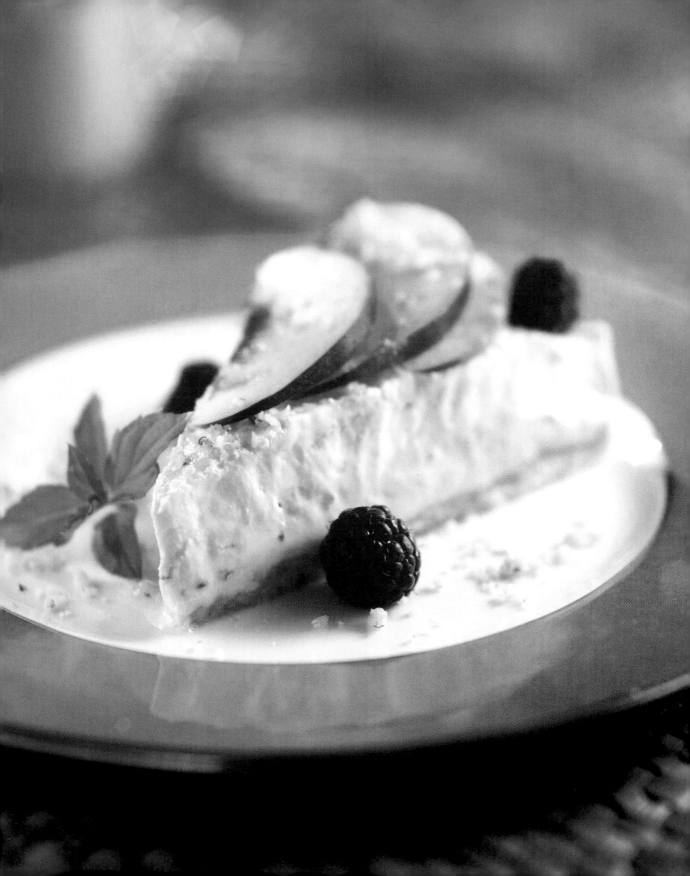

Peachy Walnut Torte

Had Marie Antoinette ever tasted this dessert, she would never had said "let them eat cake." Because the South Beach Diet is ultimately a lifestyle, an occasional indulgence in a little sugar or butter can be allowed. Just remember to savor a small piece. Enjoy!

3/4	cup English walnuts, ground
1/4	cup trans-free margarine or butter
1/4	cup sugar
2	packages (8 ounces each) reduced-fat cream cheese
1/2	cup sugar substitute
8	ounces artificially sweetened nonfat raspberry yogurt
8	ounces artificially sweetened nonfat peach yogurt
2	drops yellow food coloring
2–3	large peaches, sliced

Place 1/4 cup of the walnuts in a small bowl and set aside.

Place the remaining walnuts in another small bowl and add the margarine or butter and sugar. Mix well with a fork. Press the walnut mixture firmly into the bottom of a 8" springform pan.

In a large bowl, with an electric mixer on medium speed, beat the cream cheese and sugar substitute until smooth. Remove half of the cream cheese mixture to a medium bowl and whisk in the raspberry yogurt. Spread evenly over the walnut crust. Place in the freezer for 1 hour, or until firm.

To the remaining cream cheese mixture, add the peach yogurt and food coloring. Cover and refrigerate. When the raspberry layer has firmed, spoon the peach mixture over it. Freeze for 2 1/2 hours, or until firm.

When ready to serve, arrange the peach slices around the edge and place the reserved walnuts decoratively on top.

Makes 10 servings

NUTRITION AT A GLANCE

Per serving: 230 calories, 15 g fat, 6 g saturated fat, 8 g protein, 17 g carbohydrate, 0 g dietary fiber, 25 mg cholesterol, 200 mg sodium

Angel Meringue Dessert

This light-as-a-cloud pie will melt in your mouth.

5 egg whites, at room temperature

1/8 teaspoon salt

1/4 teaspoon cream of tartar

1/4 cup confectioners' sugar

1 teaspoon vanilla extract

2 tablespoons finely ground walnuts

1 cup low-fat frozen whipped topping, thawed

Fresh strawberries, sliced, for garnish

Mint sprigs, for garnish

Preheat the oven to 275°F.

Cover a baking sheet with parchment paper and coat the parchment paper with cooking spray.

In a large bowl, with an electric mixer on high speed, beat the egg whites and salt until soft peaks form. Gradually sprinkle in the cream of tartar and then the confectioners' sugar, 2 tablespoons at a time, beating well after each addition. Add the vanilla extract and beat until shiny peaks form. Fold in the walnuts.

Form the mixture into a 7" circle on the parchment paper.

Bake for 1 hour, or until light golden. Turn off the oven and let the meringue cool with the door open. Remove from the parchment and store in an airtight container or place on a serving plate. Top with the whipped topping and garnish with the strawberries and mint.

Makes 4 servings

NUTRITION AT A GLANCE

Per serving: 110 calories, 5 g protein, 11 g carbohydrates, 3 1/2 g fat, 1 1/2 g saturated fat, 0 mg cholesterol, 0 g dietary fiber, 140 mg sodium

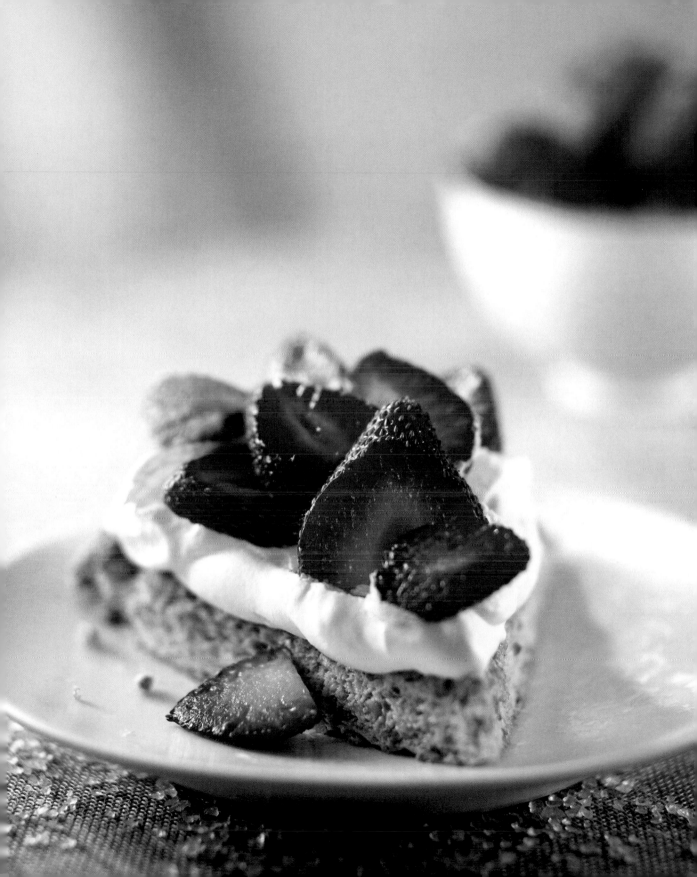

Chocolate Pie with Crispy Peanut Butter Crust

Treat yourself to some chocolate with this easy-to-make pie. The crust, made of toasted-rice cereal, is a crunchy touch that nicely complements the smooth pie.

3 tablespoons unsweetened natural peanut butter

2 cups toasted-rice cereal

1 package (1 1/2 ounces) sugar-free reduced-calorie instant chocolate pudding mix

2 cups fat-free milk

Coat an 8" or 9" pie plate with cooking spray.

In a saucepan over low heat, warm the peanut butter until melted. Remove from the heat and stir in the cereal. Press the cereal mixture into the bottom and up the side of the pie plate. Freeze for 1 hour.

Prepare the pudding according to the package directions, using the milk. Immediately pour the pudding into the prepared pie crust. Refrigerate for at least 1 hour before serving.

Makes 8 servings

NUTRITION AT A GLANCE

Per serving: 100 calories, 2 1/2 g fat, 1/2 g saturated fat, 4 g protein, 16 g carbohydrate, 0 g dietary fiber, 0 mg cholesterol, 170 mg sodium

Chocolate-Swirled Cheesecake

Cheesecake has long been an American favorite. You'll love this South Beach version, with its tantalizing swirl of semi-sweet chocolate. If you're comfortably into Phase 3, feel free to drizzle a tablespoon of semi-sweet chocolate chips on top for a crunchy garnish.

1/2	cup low-fat graham-cracker crumbs
3	cups reduced-fat ricotta cheese
4	eggs
1/2	cup sugar
1/2	cup sugar substitute
1/3	cup fat-free evaporated milk
2 1/2	squares (1 ounce each) semi-sweet chocolate, melted

Preheat the oven to 325°F.

Coat a 9" springform pan with cooking spray. Sprinkle the bottom of the pan with the cracker crumbs.

In a large bowl, with an electric mixer on medium speed, beat the cheese until light and fluffy. Add the eggs, sugar, sugar substitute, and milk and beat for 4 minutes, or until the mixture is smooth. Pour 2 cups of the batter into a small bowl and beat the melted chocolate into it.

Pour the plain batter into the prepared pan. Top with the chocolate batter. Using a knife, swirl the batters to create a marbled effect. Place the pan inside a larger one filled with 1" water.

Bake for 45 minutes, or until the edges are lightly browned and the center is nearly set. Cool on a rack for 30 minutes, then refrigerate overnight.

Makes 12 servings

NUTRITION AT A GLANCE

Per serving: 190 calories, 7 g fat, 3 1/2 g saturated fat, 8 g protein, 24 g carbohydrate, 0 g dietary fiber, 85 mg cholesterol, 100 mg sodium

Flourless Chocolate Cake with Almonds

It's rare that a person doesn't love chocolate cake. This is a flourless version that looks somewhat flat after baking, but the taste is far from it! Almonds and bittersweet chocolate provide a rich, decadent taste in every bite.

2 tablespoons trans-free margarine or unsalted butter

1 tablespoon unsweetened cocoa powder

1/2 cup blanched almonds

1/2 cup sugar

3 ounces bittersweet chocolate

1/2 cup fat-free sour cream

1/4 cup sugar substitute

2 egg yolks

1 teaspoon vanilla extract

1/4 teaspoon almond extract (optional)

5 egg whites, at room temperature

1/4 teaspoon salt

1 tablespoon toasted slivered almonds (optional)

Preheat the oven to 350°F.

Generously coat a 9" springform pan with 2 teaspoons of the margarine or butter and dust with the cocoa powder. (Don't tap out the excess cocoa; leave it in the pan.)

In a food processor, combine the blanched almonds with 2 tablespoons of the sugar. Process until finely ground.

In the top of a double boiler over barely simmering water, melt the chocolate and the remaining 4 teaspoons butter, stirring occasionally, until smooth. Remove from the heat. Place the chocolate mixture in a large bowl. Add the almond mixture, sour cream, sugar substitute, egg yolks, vanilla extract, almond extract (if using), and 1/4 cup of the remaining sugar. Stir until well-blended.

In a large bowl, with an electric mixer on high speed, beat the egg whites and salt until frothy. Gradually add the remaining 2 tablespoons sugar, beating until stiff, glossy peaks form.

Stir one-quarter of the beaten whites into the chocolate mixture to lighten it. Gently fold in the remaining whites until no white streaks remain. Place in the prepared pan. Gently smooth the top.

Bake for 30 minutes, or until the cake has risen, the top is dry, and a wooden pick inserted in the center comes out with a few moist crumbs.

Place the pan on a rack and cool until warm. The cake will fall dramatically. Loosen the edges of the cake with a knife and remove the pan sides. Sprinkle with the toasted almonds, if using.

Makes 12 servings

NUTRITION AT A GLANCE

Per serving: 150 calories, 9 g fat, 0 g saturated fat, 5 g protein, 14 g carbohydrate, 1 g dietary fiber, 35 mg cholesterol, 95 mg sodium

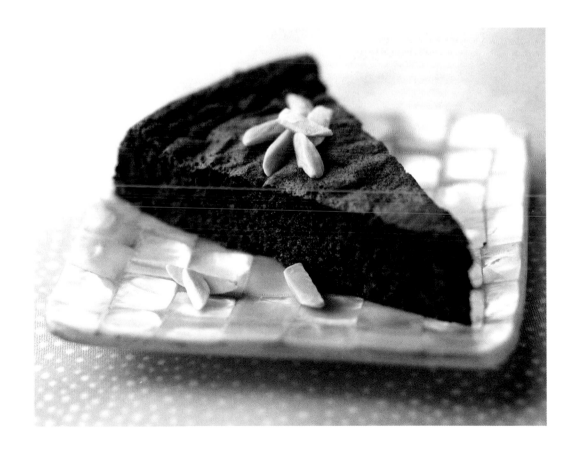

Spice Cake

It's still Phase 3, but this spice cake is a great alternative to fruit cake or gingerbread around the holidays.

1 1/2 cups whole wheat or whole grain pastry flour

1 teaspoon baking powder

1 teaspoon baking soda

1 teaspoon ground nutmeg

1 teaspoon ground cinnamon

1/2 teaspoon ground allspice

Pinch of salt

1/4 cup sugar substitute

1/2 cup sugar

2 eggs, beaten

3/4 cup unsweetened applesauce

1/3 cup canola oil

Preheat the oven to 375°F.

In a large bowl, combine the flour, baking powder, baking soda, nutmeg, cinnamon, allspice, and salt.

In another large bowl, combine the sugar substitute, sugar, eggs, applesauce, and oil. Pour the egg mixture into the flour mixture and mix thoroughly. Pour into a 9" cake pan.

Bake for 45 minutes, or until a wooden pick inserted in the center comes out clean. Cool in the pan on a rack.

Makes 8 servings

NUTRITION AT A GLANCE

Per serving: 240 calories, 11 g fat, 1 g saturated fat, 5 g protein, 31 g carbohydrate, 4 g dietary fiber, 55 mg cholesterol, 250 mg sodium

New York-Style Cheesecake

Ah, cheesecake New York–style. It just doesn't get any better! So just close your eyes, and imagine capping off a delicious al fresco dinner in one of the city's best restaurants with this creamy delight.

    4 cups reduced-fat ricotta cheese
    3 eggs, separated
    2 tablespoons honey
  1/4 cup sugar substitute
    3 tablespoons cornstarch
    1 tablespoon vanilla extract
  1/3 cup low-fat graham-cracker crumbs

Preheat the oven to 350°F.

In a large bowl, beat the cheese until smooth. Stir in the egg yolks, honey, sugar substitute, cornstarch, and vanilla extract, mixing until thoroughly combined.

In a medium bowl, whip the egg whites with clean beaters for 2 minutes, or until soft peaks form. Fold the whites into the cheese mixture.

Coat a 9" springform pan with cooking spray and cover the bottom with the cookie crumbs. Pour the cheese mixture into the pan.

Bake for 30 to 40 minutes, or until golden and set.

Makes 10 servings

NUTRITION AT A GLANCE

Per serving: 180 calories, 6 g fat, 3 g saturated fat, 10 g protein, 18 g carbohydrate, 0 g dietary fiber, 90 mg cholesterol, 125 mg sodium

Light as a Feather Lemon Cookies

Be a smart cookie and make some dough—this dough!
These lemony baked treats are a fitting final touch
to any meal.

1 1/4	cups cake flour
3	tablespoons sugar substitute
3	tablespoons confectioners' sugar
1 1/2	tablespoons grated lemon peel
1	teaspoon baking powder
1/4	cup trans-free margarine
1	egg, beaten
1	tablespoon fresh lemon juice
1	tablespoon confectioners' sugar for dusting

In a food processor, combine the flour, sugar substitute, 3 tablespoons confectioners' sugar, lemon peel, and baking powder. Add the margarine and pulse on and off until coarse crumbs form. Add the egg and lemon juice and process just until a dough forms.

Form the dough into a ball and wrap it in plastic wrap. Refrigerate the dough for at least 1 hour, or until firm.

Preheat the oven to 350°F.

Coat a baking sheet with cooking spray.

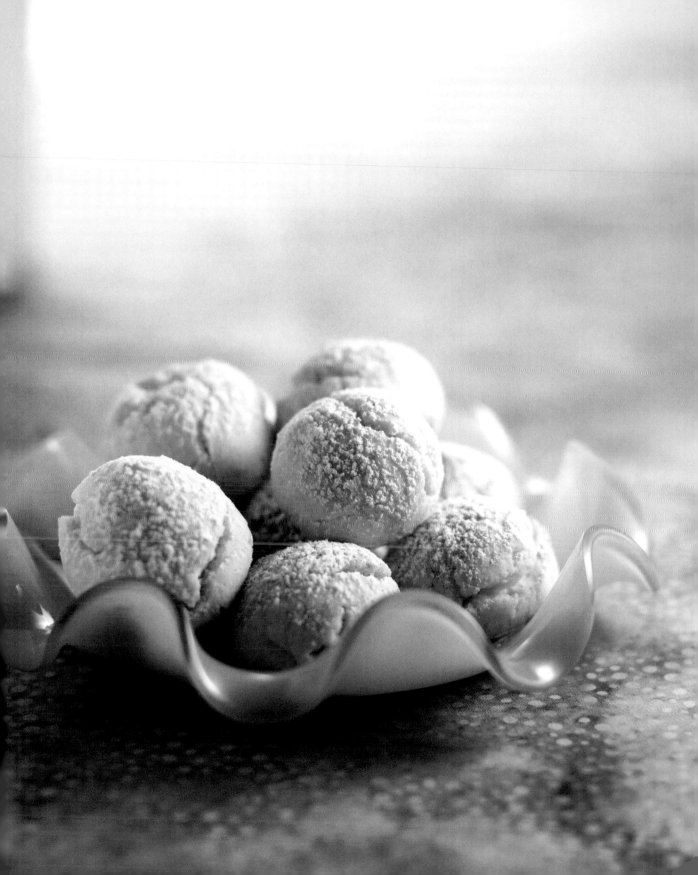

Shape the dough into 1" balls and place them 1" apart on the prepared baking sheet.

Bake for 10 minutes, or until the cookies are golden. Remove the cookies from the baking sheet and dust them with the 1 tablespoon confectioners' sugar. Cool on a rack.

Makes 24 cookies

NUTRITION AT A GLANCE
Per cookie: 50 calories, 2 g fat, 0 g saturated fat, 1 g protein, 8 g carbohydrate, 0 g dietary fiber, 10 mg cholesterol, 40 mg sodium

Lemon Cheesecake

Cheesecake was one of man's earliest produced treats, and may the tradition continue.

> 1 1/2 pounds reduced-fat ricotta cheese
>
> 1 1/2 pounds 1% reduced-fat cottage cheese
>
> 1/2 cup + 1 tablespoon sugar substitute
>
> 1/2 cup sugar
>
> 2 teaspoons cornstarch
>
> Juice of 1 lemon
>
> 2 teaspoons flour
>
> 5 eggs
>
> 3 teaspoons vanilla extract
>
> 1 1/2 cups fat-free sour cream

Preheat the oven to 400°F.

Coat a 10" springform pan with cooking spray and line the sides with a double layer of 6"-wide (high) waxed paper.

In a large bowl, with an electric mixer on medium speed, blend the ricotta cheese, cottage cheese, 1/2 cup of the sugar substitute, and sugar until smooth. Beat in the cornstarch, lemon juice, flour, eggs, and 2 teaspoons of the vanilla extract. Pour the batter into the prepared pan.

Bake for 1 hour and 10 minutes, or until the top of the cake is brown. Turn the oven off and allow the cake to remain in the oven for 1 hour longer.

In a medium bowl, combine the sour cream, the remaining 1 tablespoon sugar substitute, and the remaining 1 teaspoon vanilla extract. Spread over the cheesecake and return to the oven for 10 minutes, or until the topping is set. Refrigerate for 8 hours or overnight before slicing.

Makes 10 servings

NUTRITION AT A GLANCE

Per serving: 190 calories, 5 g fat, 2 1/2 g saturated fat, 16 g protein, 17 g carbohydrate, 0 g dietary fiber, 105 mg cholesterol, 330 mg sodium

New-Fashioned Peanut Butter Cookies

Here's a recipe for old-fashioned cookies with a new-fashioned South Beach flair. They're so tasty, you'll bake up batches of these cookies for the holidays—and more!

6	tablespoons trans-free margarine, softened
1/2	cup unsweetened natural creamy peanut butter, at room temperature
1/4	cup packed granulated brown sugar substitute (see the note on page 326)
1/4	cup sugar substitute
1	large egg, at room temperature, lightly beaten
1	teaspoon vanilla extract
1 1/4	cups sifted oat flour
1/4	teaspoon baking powder
3	tablespoons salted peanuts, chopped

Place an oven rack in the middle position and preheat the oven to 350°F.

In a large bowl, with an electric mixer on medium speed, beat together the margarine and peanut butter for 1 minute, or until very smooth. Add the brown sugar and sugar substitutes and beat for 2 minutes, or until well-combined and light in color. Gradually beat in the egg and vanilla extract, beating until very smooth and a little fluffy. Mix in the flour and baking powder, beating until a moist but cohesive dough forms. Stir in the peanuts.

Drop by the tablespoon about 2" apart on nonstick baking sheets. Using the tines of a fork dampened in cold water, flatten each in a cross-hatch pattern until 2" in diameter.

Bake for 15 minutes, or until golden brown. Remove to a rack to cool.

Makes 24 cookies

NUTRITION AT A GLANCE

Per cookie: 100 calories, 6 g fat, 1 1/2 g saturated fat, 3 g protein, 10 g carbohydrate, 1 g dietary fiber, 10 mg cholesterol, 65 mg sodium

CREDITS

The recipe for Artichokes in Olive Oil on page 94 and 95 is printed with permission of Antonio Ellek, owner, and Tulin Tuzel and Carla Ellek, chefs, of Pasha's.

The recipe for Casa Tua Restaurant Tuna Tartare on page 98 and 99 is printed with permission of Michele Grendene, owner, and Sergio Sigala, chef, of Casa Tua Restaurant.

The recipe for Wild Mushroom Cappuccino on page 116 and 117 is printed with permission of Shareef Malnik, owner, and Andrew Rothschild, chef, of The Forge.

The recipe for Classic Gazpacho with Avocado Crab Farci on pages 130–132 is printed with permission of Julian Serrano, executive chef of Picasso.

The recipe for Roasted Yellow Pepper Soup with Fava Beans and Teardrop Tomatoes on pages 140–142 is printed with permission of Andrea Curto-Randazzo and Frank Randazzo, owners and chefs of Talula Restaurant & Bar.

The recipes for Manhattan Clam Chowder on pages 150 and 151 and Sweet Onion Dressing on page 232 to 233 are printed with permission of Jo Ann Bass, owner, and André Bienvenu, chef, of Joe's Stone Crab.

The recipe for Shaved Fennel Salad with Seared Tuna and Parmesan on pages 174–176 is printed with permission of the Mandarin Oriental, owner, and Michelle Bernstein, chef, of Azul.

The recipe for Vegetable (Chinese Long Bean) Salad with Feta on pages 194–196 is printed with permission of Jonathan Eismann, owner and chef of Pacific Time.

The recipe for Grilled Mahi Mahi on Chopped Salad with Olive Oil Lemon Vinaigrette on pages 252 and 253 is printed with permission of Charlie Hines, managing director, and Marc Ehrler, executive chef, of Preston's at The Loews Miami Beach Hotel.

The recipes for Broiled Sea Bass Staten Island Style on pages 256 and 257 and Macaluso's Escarole and Beans on pages 434 and 435 are printed with permission of Michael D'Andrea, owner and chef of Macaluso's.

The recipe for Barbecue Salmon on pages 264–266 is printed with permission of Jeffrey Chodorow, owner, and Keyvan Behnam, chef, of China Grill.

The recipe for Shellfish in a Pot on pages 280–282 is printed with permission of Barton G. Weiss, owner, and Ted Mendez, chef, of Barton G The Restaurant.

The recipe for Grouper with Baby Bok Choy and Soy-Ginger Vinaigrette on pages 287–289 is printed with permission of Eric Ripert, owner and chef of Le Bernardin.

The recipes for Asparagus, Crabmeat, and Grapefruit Salad on pages 293–295 and Grilled Filet Mignon with Roasted Garlic and Chipolte Pepper Chimichurri on pages 379–381 are printed with permission of Smith & Wollensky restaurant group and Robert Mignola, chef, of Smith & Wollensky.

The recipe for Spanish Spice Rubbed Chicken with Mustard–Green Onion Sauce on pages 308–310 is printed with permission of Bobby Flay, owner and chef of Bolo Restaurant & Bar.

The recipe for Healthy Bird on pages 336 and 337 is printed with permission of Kevin Aoki, owner, and Hiro Terada, chef, of Doraku.

The recipe for Grilled Lamb Loin Salad with Chilled Greek Olive Ratatouille on pages 351–353 is printed with permission of Jose Vilarello and Geoffrey Cousineau, chef, of The Biltmore Hotel.

The recipe for Bolivian Spiced Pork Chops on pages 386–388 is printed with permission of Norman Van Aken, owner and chef of Norman's.

The recipe for Roasted Pork Tenderloin with Chickpeas, Roasted Peppers, and Clams on pages 394–396 is printed with permission of Rodrigo Martinez and Tim Andriola, co-owners of Timo.

The recipe for Veal Mignon on pages 399–401 is printed with permission of Jeffrey Chodorow, owner, and Claude Troisgros, chef, of Blue Door at Delano.

The recipe for Mediterranean Vegetable Risotto with Organic Short-Grain Brown Rice on pages 412–414 is printed with permission of Melanie Muss, owner, and

Russell Martoccio, chef, of Bleau View at the Fontainebleau Hilton Resort.

The recipe for Caribbean Ratatouille on pages 420 and 421 is printed with permission of Allen Susser, owner and chef of Chef Allen's.

INDEX

Note: <u>Underscored</u> page references indicate boxed text.
Boldfaced page references indicate photographs.

I

Ice cream, 41
Ice milk, 41
Insulin, 23

J

Jenkins, David, 7
Joe's Stone Crab, <u>150</u>, <u>232</u>

L

Lamb, 26
  Grilled Lamb Loin Salad
    with Chilled Greek
    Olive Ratatouille,
    <u>351–53</u>
Lemons
  Broiled Salmon with
    Creamy Lemon Sauce,
    261
  Citrus Vinaigrette, <u>294</u>
  Garlic and Lemon Grilled
    Vegetables, 440–41
  Lemon Cheesecake,
    483–84
  Light as a Feather
    Lemon Cookies,
    480–82, **481**

Lentils
  Chicken and Red Lentil
    Soup, 162–63
Limes
  Chicken with Lime
    Dressing, 306–7
  Citrus Vinaigrette, <u>294</u>
  Tiered Salad with Lime
    Dressing, 188–89
Lobster, 25
  Lobster Bisque, 159–60,
    161
  Shellfish in a Pot, <u>280–82</u>
Loews Miami Beach Hotel,
  <u>252–53</u>

M

Macaluso's, <u>256</u>, <u>434</u>
Mahi mahi
  Ceviche, 251
  Grilled Mahi Mahi on
    Chopped Salad with
    Olive Oil Lemon
    Vinaigrette, <u>252–53</u>
Mayonnaise, 19, 24, 30,
  237
Meats. *See also* Beef; Lamb;
  Pork
  fattiest cuts of, 20
  leanest cuts of, 26, 347

Mozzarella cheese *(cont.)*
Pork and Pepper Salad
with Balsamic
Vinaigrette, 190–92,
191
for snacks, 24
Whole Wheat Vegetable
Lasagna, 431–32, **433**
Muffins, 18, 57
Apple Walnut Muffins,
51–52
Soy-ous Apricot Muffins,
47–48
Wholesome Oat Muffins,
49–50
Mushrooms
Almond Perch Sauté,
283–84
Baked Portobello Caps
with Melted Goat
Cheese, 442, **443**
Barbecue Salmon,
264–66, **265**
Barley with Mushrooms,
438–39
Homestyle Green Bean
Casserole, 217–18, **219**
New Beef Burgundy,
375–76
Sausage and Cheese
Breakfast Cups, 79

Steak and Mushroom
Kebabs, 354–55
Teriyaki Mushroom Soup
with Watercress, 135
Wild Mushroom
Cappuccino, 116–17
Mustard, 19, 24, 30, 236–37
Chinese Mustard Sauce,
265
Mustard–Green Onion
Sauce, 308
South Beach Ballpark
Mustard, 243–44

N

Norman's, 386
Nuts. *See also specific nuts*
nut butters made from, 40
for snacks, 27
in South Beach Diet, 11

O

Oats and oat bran, 18, 29
Oatmeal Pancakes, 66–67
Oat Smoothie, 46
Wholesome Oat Muffins,
49–50
Obesity, 1, 5, 8–9, 11
Oils, healthy, 24, 27

Conversion Chart

These equivalents have been slightly rounded to make measuring easier.

VOLUME MEASUREMENTS

U.S.	Imperial	Metric
¼ tsp	–	1 ml
½ tsp	–	2 ml
1 tsp	–	5 ml
1 Tbsp	–	15 ml
2 Tbsp (1 oz)	1 fl oz	30 ml
¼ cup (2 oz)	2 fl oz	60 ml
⅓ cup (3 oz)	3 fl oz	80 ml
½ cup (4 oz)	4 fl oz	120 ml
⅔ cup (5 oz)	5 fl oz	160 ml
¾ cup (6 oz)	6 fl oz	180 ml
1 cup (8 oz)	8 fl oz	240 ml

WEIGHT MEASUREMENTS

U.S.	Metric
1 oz	30 g
2 oz	60 g
4 oz (¼ lb)	115 g
5 oz (⅓ lb)	145 g
6 oz	170 g
7 oz	200 g
8 oz (½ lb)	230 g
10 oz	285 g
12 oz (¾ lb)	340 g
14 oz	400 g
16 oz (1 lb)	455 g
2.2 lb	1 kg

LENGTH MEASUREMENTS

U.S.	Metric
¼"	0.6 cm
½"	1.25 cm
1"	2.5 cm
2"	5 cm
4"	11 cm
6"	15 cm
8"	20 cm
10"	25 cm
12" (1')	30 cm

PAN SIZES

U.S.	Metric
8" cake pan	20 × 4 cm sandwich or cake tin
9" cake pan	23 × 3.5 cm sandwich or cake tin
11" × 7" baking pan	28 × 18 cm baking tin
13" × 9" baking pan	32.5 × 23 cm baking tin
15" × 10" baking pan	38 × 25.5 cm baking tin (Swiss roll tin)
1½ qt baking dish	1.5 liter baking dish
2 qt baking dish	2 liter baking dish
2 qt rectangular baking dish	30 × 19 cm baking dish
9" pie plate	22 × 4 or 23 × 4 cm pie plate
7" or 8" springform pan	18 or 20 cm springform or loose-bottom cake tin
9" × 5" loaf pan	23 × 13 cm or 2 lb narrow loaf tin or pâté tin

TEMPERATURES

Fahrenheit	Centigrade	Gas
140°	60°	–
160°	70°	–
180°	80°	–
225°	105°	¼
250°	120°	½
275°	135°	1
300°	150°	2
325°	160°	3
350°	180°	4
375°	190°	5
400°	200°	6
425°	220°	7
450°	230°	8
475°	245°	9
500°	260°	–